YOGA FOR PREGNANCY AND BIRTH

A GUIDE FOR EXPECTANT PARENTS

YOGA FOR PREGNANCY AND BIRTH

by Nina Shandler and
Michael Shandler

Photographs by Rodney Polden

JOHN MURRAY

Acknowledgments

We are grateful to Baba Hari Dass for providing us with the technical understanding of yoga which led to the development of this project. To Richard Pokorney who took the original photographs of Manju's birth, to Steven Thomas for his photographic contribution, to Gurija who patiently posed for the postures, to Alan and Heather Martin who shared their pregnancy, to Rod Polden for his excellent photographs, to Roberta and Dennis Cloutier of Studio I, Southbridge, Massachusetts, for their selfless attitude and for the 25 photographs of Nina that appear in the book, to Kendra Crossen who polished our words so patiently, and to Patricia Woodruff, our editor, we offer our thanks.

CONTENTS

FOREWORD BY R. WINONA ROWAT, M.D.

The mental and physical benefits to be gained from the daily practice and discipline of yoga during pregnancy cannot be overestimated.

In a time when many technical advances are being made to help with birthing and high-risk newborns such as premies, the greatest step for better birthing would be the improvement of prenatal health. Improvement in this area would give us healthier mothers and babies and would save society and parents great, and unnecessary, expense—and heartache. All the elaborate equipment being devised cannot make up for what a woman has done, or has not done, during her nine months of pregnancy.

Yoga for Pregnancy and Birth proposes a clean, natural diet for pregnant women and emphasizes the importance of the emotional calm and centering that can be achieved through meditation. It also promotes the general body fitness and flexibility that comes from the daily practice of asanas (yoga postures). More general endurance exercises such as hiking, walking, and swimming complement the asanas and give the staying power necessary during labor.

Expectant parents are given an opportunity, through this beautiful book, to realize that everything in their lives is felt by the baby in the womb. Through the daily practice of a yoga way of life, parents and the new baby will flourish.

ABOUT THIS BOOK

Yoga for Pregnancy and Birth is about yoga in the deep and expansive sense of the word. The word *yoga* usually evokes images of people standing on their heads or touching their toes or sitting in cross-legged posture. These images are proper. Yoga is, in one sense, an exquisite system for stretching, relaxing, and strengthening the physical body.

Yoga is, however, a larger concept. In Sanskrit, the word has two common meanings: "to yoke" and "union." The translation "yoke" speaks of the aspect of yoga which is discipline. Yoga is a clearly and specifically designed system used to gain control over the mind and body through the regular practice of physical postures, breathing exercises, meditation, and positive behavior.

But if yoga were only a system of discipline and control, it would be a dry, austere method devoid of spirit. It is not. Yoga in the sense of "union" means union with God—the Supreme Consciousness that is our true self. Every time we touch the deeper aspects of our being, we are practicing yoga. Through yoga we realize that God is within us and within every living being, and thus the path to union is alive with peace, happiness, and love.

This book is about appreciating the presence of God within expectant mothers and fathers and within their babies. It is a responsible book which delineates the systems and methods of yoga while reminding the reader of the spirit behind yoga. We hope that it communicates the peace and joy that we have touched through yoga and that it will help you touch those qualities within yourself, your husband or wife, and your child.

The creation of a new life is a couple's most blessed adventure. This adventure begins with lovemaking and conception, continues with gestation, and culminates in childbirth. It is a special time when a woman carries two souls in one body and then brings the second soul into the world. It is an awesome time when a man feels himself close to the source of creation.

Pregnancy is a time to be cherished, to be deeply appreciated, a time in which peace, joy, lovingness, gratitude, and contentment can be nurtured.

These qualities are, however, not always easy to maintain. Well-intentioned relatives, books, or friends often excite an expectant mother's latent fears, insecurities, and emotional instabilities. They will tell "be careful" stories and "what if" sagas. A pregnant woman wants the best for her child; she is susceptible to such cautionary tales. Therefore, we offer this book as a practical guide through which you can find ease and touch peace inside yourself, which is the purpose of yoga.

During pregnancy, a woman has an added incentive to develop calmness and contentment—she's being calm for two. Contentment will touch the baby's as well as the mother's heart. This book will also show how to direct energy toward greater health and vitality. Not only is it essential to develop strength and stamina for labor, but it's also important to be happy and healthy while "with child."

A joyful pregnancy followed by a peaceful birth can strengthen the ties of marriage. This book is intended to be an aid to marriage as well as to pregnancy. The complexities which pregnancy brings to a marital relationship can be appreciated through the philosophical and psychological precepts and models of yoga. These precepts and models are presented throughout the book so as to be relevant to your experience as an expectant mother or father.

Labor/birth is a heightened life experience. It is one of those special times in life that will stand vividly among the memories of both parents. For the child it is an experience that will color his or her entire being. The closeness these three—mother, father, and child—share for the hours of labor and the moments of birth can bring to their ongoing relationship a love that will help them endure the minor irritations and compromises of family life. For this reason we present yogic breathing techniques for labor and make suggestions based on yogic principles for labor and birth.

We hope that the principles, practices, and photographs in this book will help you find confidence, peace, and joy during pregnancy and birth.

Nina and Michael Shandler

ORIENTATION

1

BECOMING A MOTHER: PREGNANCY

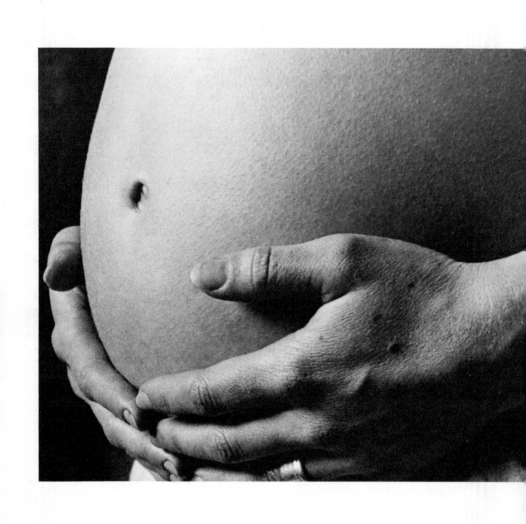

Knowing that you are going to have a baby is a great joy. But for many women, the nine months preceding the realization of that joy can be distressing because of the discomforts of morning sickness, the inevitable emotional ups and downs, and the fear of the impending labor. Sometimes it seems that pregnancy is just a "necessary evil" that must be endured in order to enjoy the fulfillment that comes with family life.

Yoga takes a different view toward pregnancy. Instead of a sometimes unpleasant prelude to a blessed event, pregnancy is itself seen as an integral part of the blessing. Yoga tells us that a woman can enjoy her pregnancy as a unique opportunity for self-development—a chance to devote herself not only to the growth of her own self, but to that of the new self taking form within her body. When a woman thinks of her pregnancy in this way, regardless of outer circumstances and the physiological and emotional changes that she faces, it becomes a period of expansion for which she is deeply grateful.

It may seem difficult to maintain this positive view during those "negative" times of your pregnancy when you feel worried or tired or queasy. But according to yoga, the way we perceive the world is conditioned by the way we think about it. As Shakespeare wrote, "There is nothing either good or bad, but thinking makes it so." Thus we have the power to make our world positive and joyful by directing our thoughts in a positive and joyful way.

In this chapter we discuss the emotional and physical changes that pregnancy brings. Understanding the sources of these changes will help you to deal with them appropriately and with confidence.

The Source of Emotional and Physical Changes

Almost as soon as conception occurs, a woman's body and emotions begin to change. The immediacy of these changes is due, in part, to a special kind of energy which becomes active in the woman's body shortly after conception. This energy, called anant vayu, is latent in all women and becomes active only during pregnancy.

Anant vayu has several functions. It affects the growth of the fetus in the womb by combining with energy from the mother's physiological processes, and at the same time it flows upward toward the heart and head of the expectant mother. Thus its functions affect both mother and child.

In the early months of pregnancy the movements of anant vayu may cause morning sickness or nausea. The body is preparing for the many physical adjustments necessary to the process of pregnancy, and the effects of this adjustment may be felt through the action of anant vayu. Once this stage is completed, nausea usually subsides.

After morning sickness has subsided, anant vayu takes on a much richer function and becomes a source of elation to the expectant mother. Now the impulse becomes easily aroused, with the result that a woman in this stage is far more sensitive than normal. Through the practice of asanas (physical postures), breathing, meditation, reading inspirational literature, and dwelling on loving, hopeful thoughts, anant vayu is activated in a balanced way and enables a pregnant woman to feel peace and happiness in abundance. This heightened susceptibility to positive feelings is the main function of anant vayu. It gives the mother, and thus the child, a sense of well-being, a precious gift from nature.

During labor, anant vayu serves to intoxicate the mother's mind so that the pain of childbirth is lessened. The depression that many women feel after giving birth is due to the subsiding of anant vayu. However, if a balanced program of yoga is continued after delivery, the change need not be so dramatic.

Anant vayu can be strengthened and stabilized by using specific methods. Yogic meditation, breathing exercises, asanas, and the development of right thinking are all designed to increase and balance the positive benefits of anant vayu. There is no doubt that if these methods are practiced regularly, this natural energy impulse will be the blessing it was intended to be.

Remedies for Morning Sickness

The discomfort of morning sickness affects a vast number of expectant mothers during the first three months of pregnancy. When I was pregnant, I found little solace in the knowledge that it would probably last "only" three months. Three hours of nausea seemed about all I could take, three days were perhaps tolerable, but three months seemed outrageous! After a couple of weeks of depression and resentment about my physical condition, I accepted the unalterable reality. I had no choice. Although my discomfort continued, my attitude changed. I became more serene. This newly acquired calm enabled me to weather the nausea in a more cheerful spirit. As a result the three months were not the eternity I had anticipated.

If morning sickness is inescapable for you too, try some of the methods to ease the discomfort which we share in this chapter, and if you are lucky you may alleviate it entirely. But if you are unable to relieve your discomfort, then your mental attitude becomes all important. The thought that in seven or eight months you will have a child to care for, cuddle, and love may bring you some resignation. Also, the realization that you are being given a chance to develop endurance and patience, qualities needed for child rearing, may help you to accept this temporary experience gracefully.

There are many cures for morning sickness. Some work for some women and not for others. All of the cures we suggest are harmless. They can and should be experimented with. If one cure works, use it. If it doesn't, try another. Good luck!

Frequent Small Meals

Many women find that eating small meals at frequent intervals helps abate nausea. Concentrate on easily digested foods such as light carbohydrates. I used to have extreme cravings for baked potatoes, even at two o'clock in the morning. After eating one I'd feel comfortable for a few hours.

Vitamin B

Nutritionists often recommend B vitamins, especially vitamin B_6. Bananas, raw pecans, wheat germ, brewer's yeast, sprouted mung beans and lentils, and all grains are foods high in B vitamins.

Salty Foods

Salty food sometimes helps ease the discomfort of nausea. Umeboshi plums (plums aged in a salt solution) and soup made from miso (soybean paste) are two macrobiotic specialties; both products can be found in health food stores. Or you might try salted crackers or vegetable broth. Greek olives were the salty treat I found most effective. I kept a good supply in the fridge and nibbled them often.

Ume Syo Kuzu

Sipped alone or used as a soup base, this delicious broth may be a pleasant way to rid yourself of discomfort. To make it you need fresh ginger root, umeboshi plums, kuzu (a vegetable root starch similar to arrowroot), and tamari soy sauce. These can be obtained at most health food stores. Grate one-quarter inch of ginger root and simmer it in two cups of water for ten minutes. Then add one umeboshi plum and a teaspoon of tamari soy sauce. Dissolve one-half teaspoon of powdered kuzu root in one tablespoon of cold water and add it to the mixture. When the kuzu has become transparent, the drink is ready.

Herbal Remedies

The following suggested herbal remedies have natural, gentle medicinal qualities and can be used without fear of harm to yourself or your baby. A remedy to be taken at the first signs of nausea may be prepared by combining equal parts of powdered cloves and powdered white poplar bark. This mixture can be sweetened with honey and taken with water, or it can be put into capsules and swallowed. A teaspoon of this mixture can be taken twice a day.

To make a treatment for vomiting, simmer one ounce of spearmint leaves and one teaspoon of powdered turkey rhubarb root *(Rheum palmatum)* in one pint of water for ten minutes in a covered container. Pour this heated mixture over one teaspoon of powdered cloves and one teaspoon of powdered cinnamon. Cover and let cool. Take one tablespoon every half hour, sweetened with honey if you like.

Fresh Air

If the air where you live is fresh, then taking short walks and breathing in pleasant smells can relieve the stagnant feeling that sometimes accompanies nausea.

Rest and Relaxation

The first three months of pregnancy should be a period of luxurious living, if possible. Treat yourself well. Catnap when you feel like it. Eat out if you enjoy it. Read your favorite literature. Go to movies. Embroider. Relieve yourself of as much emotional and physical strain as you possibly can.

Sleep Patterns

From the very beginning of pregnancy, women often find that their normal sleep patterns become drastically changed. The usual active day followed by seven or eight hours of sleep is replaced by periods of excessive daytime sleep and/or nighttime insomnia.

It is not unusual for an expectant mother to feel tired and listless during the first three months of pregnancy. Sometimes this need for sleep accompanies morning sickness. At other times, women who do not experience morning sickness do find themselves napping for long periods of time throughout the day.

During the early stages of pregnancy, the body is undergoing an adjustment which may make frequent rest necessary. Naps can rejuvenate the body and mind. At times the same or even a greater rejuvenating effect may be experienced by taking the Corpse pose (see page 94) for fifteen minutes. It is said that if this pose is done properly, the body and mind become totally relaxed, so that a few minutes of practice can replace hours of sleep.

A warning about overindulgence in sleep deserves mention, however. As long as rest is rejuvenating, it is beneficial. It is possible to sleep and rest too much, however. The body can become increasingly lethargic if unnecessary sleep becomes a habit. Sleeping out of boredom or a desire to escape just breeds more tiredness. If you do not arise from sleep or rest with increased vitality, then you probably need exercise, fresh air, social contact, or some engaging activity. Try an alternative to sleep. Perhaps your enthusiasm and energy will increase.

Generally, women find that their vitality increases after the first three months of pregnancy. You probably will become your old active self again once your body adjusts to carrying a baby inside it. At this time, it is important to become disciplined about your daily routine of breathing exercises, meditation, and yoga postures. Pregnancy, labor, and birth are emotionally and physically demanding. Meeting these challenges can be a happy venture if the mind is kept calm and the body strong.

From the fourth to the eighth month, many women become insomniacs. Your day may be filled with relaxing enjoyable activity, your mind calmly joyful—yet you are unable to sleep through the night. Don't be anxious about this seemingly "nervous" irregularity in sleep. After all, there's no reason to feel upset about being awake for a couple of hours in the night. It is quite enjoyable to practice yoga during this time. The night, especially when everyone else is asleep, is a quiet time that is particularly conducive to deep meditation, breathing exercises, or practice of asanas. Sleep after yoga practice is often very deep. The quality of sleep you get can more than make up for the lack of quantity.

The last month of pregnancy is uncomfortable for some women: they feel tired from the weight they have gained. However, by filling the first months with meditation, breathing exercises, practice of asanas, good food, and fresh air, you can ensure a more comfortable last month.

If you do feel tired, it might be due to the desire to just have your baby and to stop being a "fat lady." This "sick of being pregnant" feeling is especially true for first-time mothers because a first child often arrives late. It's quite normal for a first pregnancy to be as much as two weeks overdue. That two weeks can seem like an eternity. Very likely you will be asked several times a day if you've gone into labor yet. You may wish it would happen just so you won't have to answer the phone and say no even one more time!

Whatever your reason for tiredness in this last month, respond to it by doing what feels best. Sleep if that helps. Exercise if it invigorates you. Try to maintain a disciplined routine of meditation and yoga practices even if it is necessary to limit the postures you use. Labor is approaching, it *will* come, and you will need to draw on your resources of physical and emotional strength. Maintenance of these strengths will make your task easier.

The last few days before labor are often marked by a burst of energy and enthusiasm. You might suddenly decide to start cleaning the whole house, or swim for hours, or even go ice-skating! I did asanas for about three hours the afternoon before my daughter was born. On the previous day I had decided to walk around New York instead of taking the subway. By the time my shopping was finished, I had walked about fifty blocks without even noticing it! This surge of energy seems to be one of nature's wonderful gifts, enabling a mother to fully appreciate the birth of her child.

Increased Awareness of the Senses

The activity of the senses is heightened during pregnancy. Tastes, smells, sounds, sights, and sensations are noticed more acutely. In fact, increased sensitivity to smells is often a symptom of pregnancy.

During the first three months smells can be a cure or a cause of nausea. Fresh, sweet-smelling air can make you feel better. But even a slightly disagreeable smell can irritate an already uneasy stomach. A friend of ours asked her husband to wash and scour a frying pan repeatedly because its aroma of curry disturbed her. No matter how hard he scrubbed, she could still smell the residue. Finally, they stopped using the pan.

The increased sensitivity of smell is very noticeable to the pregnant woman because her physical reaction is so strong. Nevertheless her other senses are also heightened. The sensitivity is, in part, the reason she has strong cravings for certain foods and is repelled by others.

This pattern of having extreme desires and distastes carries over into other areas of life while a woman is pregnant. You will probably find yourself preoccupied with your environment. You may want to paint your whole house different colors, except for one room which you absolutely love. Your sensitivity to sight is the cause. Colors, room arrangements, cleanliness, dirt, buildings, even nature—all come under the scrutiny of your critical eye. The same is true of sounds. Music is soothing or energizing or grating. Birds singing in the morning now calm your mind and make you feel happy, whereas before you never noticed them. The sound of traffic you blocked out before now keeps you awake. Your sensitivity affects your reactions to things felt and touched. The gentle rain on your face, the feel of a cat's fur, the touch of soft clothing, are noticed and enjoyed. Likewise, unpleasant sensations cause unpleasant emotions.

The increase in sense awareness can seem both a blessing and a curse. It's simultaneously a source of pleasure and pain. There is no way to escape the discomfort of disagreeable sights, sounds, sensations, and smells while still maintaining the enjoyment of pleasant sights, sounds, sensations, and smells. For the same sensitivity that allows us to experience pleasure makes us aware of pain also.

In yoga, one of the aims of meditation is to reach a state called pratyahara in which the mind remains calm despite any outward stimulant, whether painful or pleasurable. Instead of directing attention to the external objects of the senses, the meditator centers his or her consciousness on the source of perception within. Heat, cold, noise, hunger, and smells cannot disturb the tranquility of the mind thus concentrated within itself. Pratyahara is an advanced stage of yoga practice; yet everyone has experienced this withdrawal of the senses to some degree.

There is an old story from India which illustrates this kind of concentration. A yogi clothed in the traditional robes of a holy man was sitting by the roadside practicing meditation. He sat with eyes closed, perfectly straight, in full lotus position. He had not moved for many hours. Hurrying along the road came a housewife carrying on her head a basket of food she had bought at the marketplace. As she rushed by, her sari lightly brushed the meditator's body. He arose indignantly and reproached her for disturbing his meditation. She responded apologetically, saying, "I was thinking of my husband. I'm returning home after several hours away from him. My mind was so absorbed in thoughts of him that I did not even see you. Forgive me."

When this story is told, the question follows: Whose meditation was deeper—the yogi's or the woman's?

We have all experienced this kind of absorption in thought when we are, say, preoccupied about something and all else goes unnoticed. One purpose of meditation is to develop such absorption in the thought of God, love, or peace that the power of the senses which leads us to all kinds of distractions and unnecessary attachments becomes temporarily broken. Gradually, as this ability to concentrate inwardly is strengthened, pleasant or unpleasant sensations lose their ability to cause pain or pleasure. This process helps one to develop equanimity and contentment in the face of changing circumstances.

The increased awareness of the senses can provide the pregnant woman with an incentive for developing the meditative state of mind. The discomforts she perceives through the senses are a vivid reminder of the need to find happiness from an internal source of contentment and assurance rather than from erratic, uncontrollable happenings in the external environment. It is, in a sense, a sign of effective meditation to be able to be happy even when other conditions are unpleasant to the senses. To experience this is to really feel the heart of yoga.

Food: Desire Is Necessity

Pregnancy is marked by extreme desires. Women are strongly attracted to or repulsed by everything from colors to their husbands. Food also comes under the scrutiny of a woman's strongly felt urges.

After the fourth month of pregnancy, the desires of the mother reflect, in addition to her own needs, the needs of the baby growing inside her (see page 123, "The Fourth Month"). During the first three months a pregnant woman's urges are mainly caused by her own physical need. The mother's body, adjusting to carrying a baby, demands nutritional and stabilizing foods during this time. A pregnant woman may often crave carbohydrates and salty food. She may also want chocolate or ice cream, but this is probably a desire for the enjoyment of tasting these foods, not a requirement for the health of her body.

But in the fourth month, the character of the baby changes. Now, in addition to her own needs and desires, the pregnant woman experiences the baby's desires as her own. She may find herself wanting foods she never thought of eating—ice-cream sodas, eggs, meat, pudding, eggplant. It can be

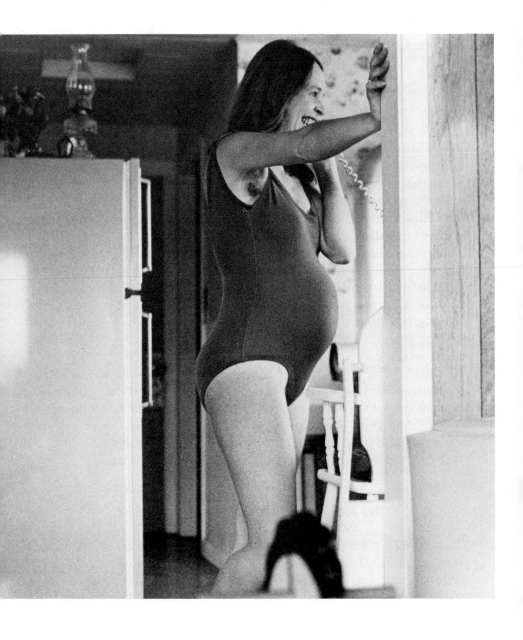

surprising to a mother how obsessed she becomes with certain foods. These obsessions are directly related to the baby's need to experience certain tastes and smells. According to yoga, these cravings should be satisfied, for they are necessary to the healthy development of the baby. (See chapter 7 for a detailed discussion of diet during pregnancy.)

The Nesting Instinct

It is said the ancient yogis learned postures by observing the behavior of animals over long periods of time. They learned to understand basic, natural ways to achieve health by watching how animals responded to sickness and stress. They then applied these principles to themselves and achieved greater health, vitality, strength, and peace of mind. It was understood that animals instinctively respond to their physical needs with the most natural and beneficial remedies.

Observing animals can also help us understand an expectant human mother's needs. When a bird expects a baby, it builds a nest. Mice find a cozy home before giving birth. Most animals settle into a home when they are about to produce young. A woman experiences the same instinctual need when she is expecting a child. Even women who tend to be ''gypsies'' experience a need for security and stability during pregnancy. A home is a natural need for a pregnant woman.

If a stable home is not provided during pregnancy, a woman may be much more susceptible to emotions of insecurity. She may worry about money, her marriage, her impending motherhood. These fears seem to subside after the birth of the child. Even if your life style necessitates frequent moves, try to remain stable for the nine months of pregnancy. It will make the time of pregnancy and the birth of your child a less stressful experience.

The Need for Quietness and Solitude

Whether you are settled into a stable home or are in a period of flux during pregnancy, it is helpful to have periods of aloneness. Tuning in to the child inside you sometimes requires delicacy and quietness. Breathing slowly, reading quietly aloud, rocking in a rocking chair, sitting by a fire, listening to music are all experiences you share with your unborn child. It takes being alone to touch these spaces of conscious communication with your baby. If you crave solitude during your pregnancy, then by all means do fulfill this need. In a way, it is your baby saying, "Mommy, I need attention."

These times of peace and solitude will help to stabilize your emotions. Pregnant women are notoriously emotional. Within your being you are carrying two souls, two hearts, two sets of desires. Small wonder that feelings are so extreme during pregnancy!

Sexual Desire: Attraction, Repulsion, Indifference

Among the most disconcerting experiences during pregnancy are the transformations in a woman's sexual desires. These transformations do not take one particular form. It's not possible to predict what set of changes will affect an expectant mother during a particular period of pregnancy.

Sexual desire may have a variety of sources. It may be motivated by a strong reproductive urge, a need for the enjoyment of sexual gratification or for emotional release, a desire for intimacy, or a need for personal affirmation. For most of us, sex is motivated by a combination of these sources. The combination varies from time to time. Sometimes our need for affirmation is greater than our desire to reproduce. Yet, at another time, our desire to have a child may be a very strong motivation. Most of us don't analyze our motivations when we desire lovemaking. We want sex and we respond to that need. We understand our desire because it has become familiar to us. If we've been married for some time, our sexual relationship has likely fallen into a particular pattern which we are now quite used to.

Pregnancy often throws that pattern out completely. For example, immediately after conception, I lost my desire to make love. This loss of sexual desire is quite common in many women. Perhaps they are dominated by a desire for children and feel temporarily satisfied once that desire is gratified.

Other women, however, experience heightened sexual desire and increased enjoyment of sex. Perhaps they are motivated by a need for closeness or affirmation while pregnant. Still other women feel extremes of attraction or repulsion. When they feel sexual desire it is a stronger and more immediate need than they normally felt before they were pregnant. But when they are not feeling desirous, it is impossible to seduce them. They feel repulsed by the thought, or the touch.

If sexual desire were a solitary activity, with no repercussions for anyone else, these changes would be of little consequence. But since your desire, or lack of it, will necessarily affect your relationship with your husband, it is

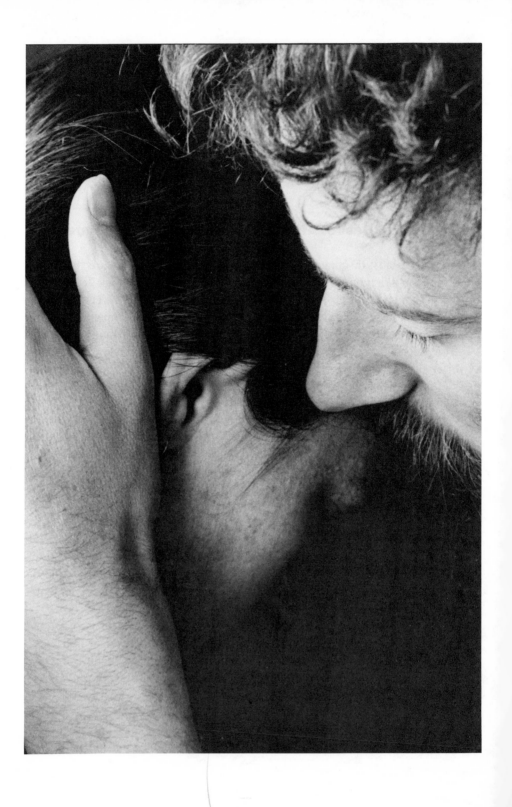

important to understand these changes in your sexual relationship—and to learn to use them as an opportunity for heightened communication.

Understanding Your Husband's Dilemma

The sexual changes a woman experiences during pregnancy may be most difficult for a man to understand and appreciate. For a married couple, sex is an expression of their unity and intimacy. If a woman becomes less interested or more demanding or generally more erratic sexually, then a husband quite naturally may feel confused. He may feel rejected, or as if he were just an instrument used to satisfy your whims. The knowledge that your changes are due to your pregnancy and have nothing to do with him or your love for him is of little consolation. Your husband's natural human need for closeness and understanding continues whether or not you're pregnant. A pregnant wife should therefore make an extra effort to empathize with her husband's point of view. He may be centered and secure in himself most of the time, but there are odd moments when his guard is down.

Giving first is a very important concept in building a relationship. If both partners in a relationship are always waiting for the other to be kind or considerate or to surrender first, then real giving will never begin. On the other hand, when one always tries to surrender first, every day is filled with a wonderful quality of love and harmony. At no other time is this ability to love first more crucial and more challenging than during pregnancy. It is crucial because pregnancy is the prelude to having a larger family. Every couple needs a continually renewing and expanding foundation of harmony to provide a loving atmosphere for their children, as well as themselves, to grow in.

During pregnancy you face the challenge of coping with your emotional and physical changes while, at the same time, learning to empathize more and more with your husband. This is one reason why pregnancy is such a wonderful opportunity to learn selfless love and surrender.

2

A CHAPTER FOR HUSBANDS: ON UNDERSTANDING YOGA AS UNION

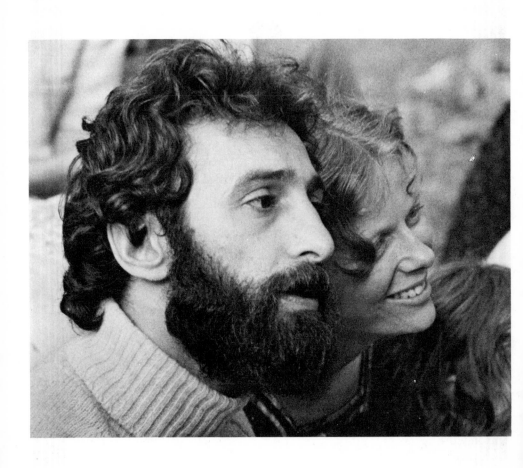

As a husband and father, I know how difficult it is to appreciate the depth of the yearning in a woman to have a baby. True, a man has a yearning for children too, but somehow it is different, for it is the woman who has the experience of carrying a new life in her own body, of bearing and nursing the newborn child. So when your wife conceives, whether it is for the first, second, or fifth time, it is always an event that will change her substantially. You, as a man, will be called upon to change too, though your changes will come more in response to the miracle taking place within your wife than purely from your own self. Truly, as yoga claims, man and woman are both pregnant together, and they have complementary roles to play in bringing a child into this world.

If you've never understood or appreciated the idea of a quantum leap, the time of pregnancy demonstrates it extremely well. You, the husband and father, will be urged to respond to your wife's pregnancy with an intensity you may seldom have experienced. From the basic demands of your wife for comfort and security, through the gamut of your interpersonal emotions, to the deepest mutual wonder at creation, both you and your wife will be pushed, prodded, tested, and required to respond.

Books are helpful when one is involved in such a process because they can provide maps of experiences that point the way. Having been students of yoga for several years, we naturally looked to the available yoga resources for the information we needed for this stage of our journey. While we found aspects of the information we needed in different places, we found no single comprehensive source we could refer to. This was frustrating, but at the same time we realized that we were involved in a transcultural experiment. The teachings of yoga and Eastern spirituality in general were being transplanted to America and we, with hundreds of thousands of others, were not only the guinea pigs in the experiment, but in some ways the experimenters as well. It was at this stage that we resolved to keep records of our experiment to share with others similarly involved.

I must say, though, that the spirit of yoga very often gets lost in technical descriptions of postures, breathing techniques, and meditations. We felt that to fully appreciate this system, to give it greater context, we should try to share a few basic yogic thoughts with the reader. The reason this is brought up here in a chapter for husbands is that from the point of view of yoga, the husband's responsibility in the pregnancy he and his wife are involved in is so great. We very much want to encourage the participation of the husband in the process of his wife's pregnancy, and perhaps a deeper discussion of yoga would be helpful in that regard.

Yoga is much more than a physical health system. It is an exquisitely articulated way of conscious living that involves learning to change the viewpoint of the mind so that human endeavors become an expression of spiritual ideals. The process by which this is achieved is called sadhana in Sanskrit, and it involves work with the whole being—the body, mind, and emotions.

This book focuses primarily upon the yoga exercises that a woman should practice during her pregnancy—her sadhana. The husband's perspective is very different and yet essential to the well-being of his wife and baby, indeed, to the harmonious formation of his family.

What is the husband's sadhana during his wife's pregnancy? It is based on the foremost yoga precept, that of selflessness. In a nutshell, one must develop an attitude in which he does not think of how he wants others to love him; instead, he thinks of how he can love them. If one feels that he is not loved enough—this is a sign that he must love more. What follows is a discussion of how this precept can be applied during pregnancy in the pursuit of harmonious living between husband and wife, the foundation of a spiritual family.

A Yoga Model for the Expectant Couple

We surrender our natures and our entire beings into each other. We accept our responsibilities and will be true to one another in this life and all future lives. We are one self operating in two bodies and we are married forever.

The Marriage Vow of Yoga

The essence of yoga is harmony. In marriage, harmony means the complementary interaction on all levels between husband and wife. Agreements are made either consciously or subconsciously as to who will play what role; where there is no agreement, strife results. Marriage is often difficult, for one's expectations are seemingly endlessly tested or probed, and during pregnancy, with its unexpected variables, one can be pushed to the limits. The next section provides an explanation of some of the variables that will arise during pregnancy, presented particularly for the husband's understanding.

Essential to this explanation is the concept of the chakras. The word *chakra* means an energy center. According to yoga, there are seven main energy centers in the human being, each of which is responsible for a physical, emotional, psychological, or spiritual aspect of being.

First and Second Chakras: The Preservation and Sexual Centers

The first center deals with the preservation-of-life instinct. It is the most basic of all human instincts and arises powerfully during pregnancy, becoming increasingly strong the nearer a woman gets to giving birth, and often lasting for several years thereafter.

This chakra's demands are quite simple: a warm, stable, and pleasant environment in which the mother-to-be can gestate peacefully. In short, your wife will be in need of a place she can call home, a place where she feels good, relaxed enough to endure morning sickness, to enjoy the afternoon sleeps that may become a part of her pregnancy, a place where she can marvel at the miracle taking place within her own body. These needs are basic, and their satisfaction is primarily the husband's responsibility.

The second chakra deals with the sexual drives and reproductive forces in the human being. There is little question that after conception your sexual relationship with your wife will change. Often a woman's sexual drive during gestation and while nursing becomes quite reduced.

The reason for this reduction in sexual drive is that during a normal monthly cycle (when a woman is not pregnant), the sexual center in a woman has two basic functions: (1) internal preparation for reproduction, and (2) the production of the vital energy in a woman's body that contributes to her health and vitality. During pregnancy a woman's internal preparation for reproduction is fully engaged, further immediate reproduction becoming impossible, and where her sexual fluids were once providing only for her own health and vitality, they now contribute to the growth and health of her baby as well.

With the understanding of what is occurring in your wife's sexual cycle, your characteristic sexual expectations can more easily be adjusted. The sexual act should be only at your wife's invitation during this time, as she is more in touch with her own internal processes and instinctively knows the appropriate responses.

In the Jewish and Hindu religions, sexual relations between husband and wife are regulated according to the woman's cycle. These regulations can shed some light on the sexual relationship during pregnancy as well. According to these religions, while the woman menstruates, and for seven days after the cessation of blood flow, husband and wife should abstain from intercourse. They are encouraged to develop their emotional, mental, and spiritual relationship during this time, complementing their understanding and appreciation of each other so that when it is once more time for physical union they are already emotionally, mentally, and spiritually attuned. Thus, there is a monthly reunion in this system. Similarly, during pregnancy, the emphasis on sex in your relationship should relaxedly be expanded into other areas of harmony you may seldom give importance to.

Third Chakra: The Vital Center

The third chakra is responsible for health and vitality in a human being. Your wife's good health and vitality are paramount during her pregnancy; a pregnant woman feels infinitely better during the pregnancy if she is really strong and healthy. Not only this, the energies required in the actual birth process are phenomenal, and a woman simply must be fit.

The development of the vital center, though, is something more than just a physical phenomenon. Health and vitality translate into strength of will, perseverance, and determination, psychological qualities that in a sense not only prepare a woman for actual delivery but create an auspicious environment for the baby in her womb, your child, to grow up in.

This is where you come in. It is your unbounded enthusiasm and encouragement that are going to be the strongest supports for your wife in her daily practices. Share with her in this process, and remember how much your support counts. Encourage her to do her daily program, and by all means join her.

You can also play a very direct part in helping your wife to develop her vitality by sharing a variety of physical treats with her. Here are a few ideas:

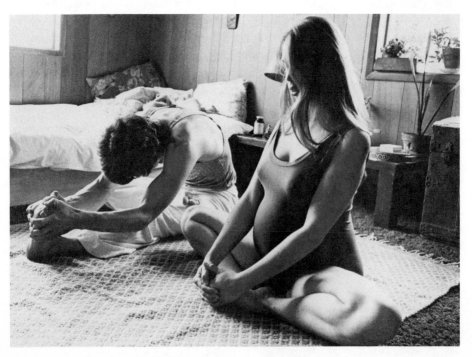

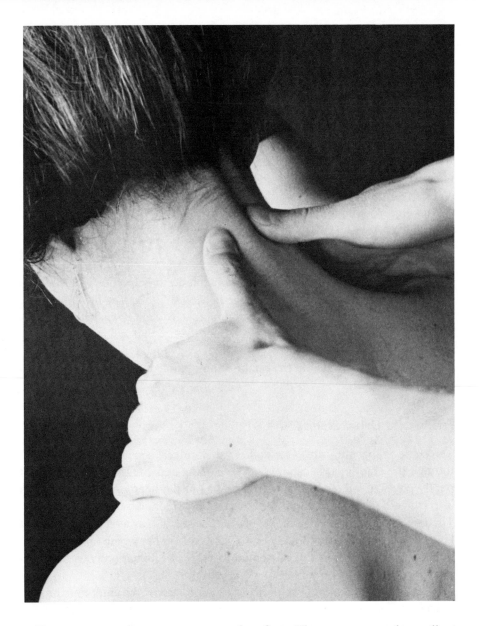

Foot massage: Learn to massage her feet. There are several excellent books that explain the location of the nerves in the feet, which, when manipulated and massaged in very simple ways, help immensely in toning up the entire system. But do be very sensitive to the feedback your wife gives you about her comfort or discomfort during a foot massage. Trust her knowledge of her own body.

Head and neck rubs: I have learned over the years that if I am calm and centered, I can help my wife to relax and find her own center by giving her a neck and head rub. It is said that if one can relax the nape of the neck, the area where the neck joins the skull, then the entire system can be relaxed. At times during pregnancy, for reasons both apparent and unapparent, your wife may become anxious or upset, and you can do her and your baby the most wonderful favor by helping them in this way. Remember the mother and baby are not separate.

Walking: Walking is great exercise for a pregnant woman. She gets fresh air and exercise and, often by just walking in a beautiful place, her whole frame of mind improves. Take walks with your wife—they'll probably do you some good too.

There are hundreds of other things you can do to help your wife become more vital, one of which is to encourage her to stick to a good diet. But more than anything else, it is your understanding that you and your wife are pregnant together that will provide a large part of the fire that will make your wife glow with good health. In turn, your child, growing day by day inside her, will be healthy and develop the qualities any father would be proud to pass on to his children.

Fourth and Fifth Chakras: The Emotional Centers

The emotional centers are often called "the bridge" because a human being, through the emotions, is capable of developing and communicating beyond purely physical values to the unseen realms of the heart. A human being is also capable of intense emotional frustration, which can result in neurosis. The important thing to realize during pregnancy is that every emotion that your wife feels is passed directly on to your child in her womb, and therefore her emotional good health is essential to your child's harmonious development.

Yoga gives much attention to the cultivation of positive emotions through exercises that specifically work with the heart. Singing and dancing to devotional songs and other activities that give expression to the heart are designed to open the emotional centers. During pregnancy the emotional side of a woman is particularly keen, and a husband can be a wonderful support to his wife during this time by understanding her sensitivity. Give every encouragement to your wife to develop uplifting emotions. This kind of support will help your wife's spirit to soar and will have a wonderful effect upon your child in her womb.

One way to share in cultivating upliftment is by reading inspiring thoughts or stories aloud to your wife. Any thoughts which touch the heart, create awe, or inspire devotion or creativity are beneficial and are doubly enhanced by sharing.

At times, though, your wife may feel emotionally upset. As far as we are able to ascertain, this is par for the course: it happens. At such times your role as a husband must really be one of compassion and support. Swallow your pride, accept the situation, and do whatever is appropriate to help your wife to come through the upheaval with a minimum of fuss.

The Sixth Chakra: The Mental Center

What we call the "mind" yoga has classified as the sixth center, second to the highest chakra in the human being. Since it is a very vast subject, we will here go into only some simple aspects about the mind that are important to consider during pregnancy.

According to yoga, it is through the mind that we create the heaven or hell that we call our lives. Our thoughts bring us with certainty to a life of beauty and harmony, or a life of negativity and fear. Yoga goes on to say that it is within the power of every human being to eradicate negative and destructive thoughts by cultivating positive thought forms and by developing good habits.

The habitual ways a person has of thinking, deep seated in his or her psyche, are called samskaras in Sanskrit. In the later stages of development in the womb before birth, the young child readily absorbs the samskaras of his parents, an unavoidable fact of life. At this stage the highest service we can perform for our children is to work on changing our own negativity. This can't be done overnight, for the mind is attached to its habitual thoughts and tendencies, but by working on dissolving our own habitual negativity, we give our children a greater opportunity to grow into clear and open human beings themselves.

The tools which yoga uses for working with the mind increase the ability of the mind to concentrate inwardly. Eventually such concentration allows the waves of mental activity to subside, and the mind becomes as calm as a peaceful lake. Life then becomes a joyous and positive expression. A couple can do much to support each other in attaining peace of mind. They can act as pillars of strength, intelligently guiding each other and feeding each other enthusiasm for their pilgrimage together. With such an example before them, it is easy for children to "catch on" and begin their own conscious evolution from a very early age. We teach best by example.

The Seventh Chakra: The Spiritual Center

Although yoga is very much concerned with the harmonization of the six lower chakra functions which we have just described, the main goal of yoga is to awaken the spiritual center. This chakra or center is the seat of love and peace. At this level of consciousness there is nothing to disturb blissful enjoyment of the Infinite; one who has attained this level, while still able to live "normally," is no longer affected by the imperfections and troubles of life.

According to yoga, two qualities are necessary prerequisites to this blissful calm. First we must develop a complete lack of self-concern, and second we must surrender to the inevitable pains and pleasures of life. Most of us have experienced brief moments when these two qualities have predominated, and our usual habits and preoccupations have been set aside. Certainly such moments stand out in the memory as deeply spiritual experiences.

The birth of a child can trigger such a temporary spiritual state in both the father and the mother, if they are well prepared. A mother instinctively knows that the baby's need to be born is her first concern, and if she obeys her deeper instincts she can surrender completely to the process of giving birth. Consequently, although she experiences the pain of labor, she also experiences a love and peace utterly unaffected by the process taking place in her body. If the husband gives himself to the needs of his wife so that she may experience as much physical, mental, and emotional support as possible, he will trigger in himself a peace and fulfillment that are not marred by the difficulties of the birth experience. If the husband and wife are able to make this psychological and emotional "jump," their baby will be born in a deeply spiritual atmosphere.

Although parents will inevitably "come down" from such a lofty experience, the birth of a child nonetheless can be a vivid reminder of the real goal of yoga. Then the attitudes necessary to sustain "life in the spirit" can be developed with greater enthusiasm and with a clear idea of the peace and love we all desire.

YOGA
PRACTICES

3

RIGHT LIVING: THE BASIS OF YOGA PRACTICE

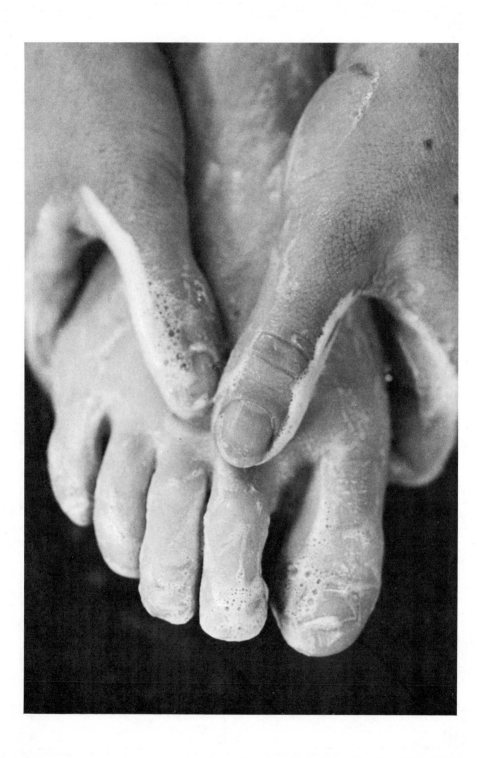

All spiritual paths have as their basis a moral way of life. The Ten Commandments of Judaism and the simple teachings of Jesus Christ are Western models for right living. Yoga also has guidelines for applying the basic principle of love—love of God, love of self, love of creation, love of neighbor—to our daily existence. These guidelines for living are restraints (yama) and observances (niyama). In introducing these guidelines for daily living, our purpose is to familiarize the reader with an aspect of yoga that is little known in our culture and yet is extremely important to understand before beginning the yoga practice of asanas, breathing, and meditation.

In its essence, yoga is based on a very personal psychology of "right attitude" in word, thought, and deed, which is the very foundation of yoga as a spiritual path. This psychology of right attitude includes such principles as noninjury, nonlying, nonstealing, noncollecting, moderation in sex, cleanliness, contentment, self-discipline, right company, and surrender. The more popularized practices of yoga—breathing exercises, meditation, and asanas—are complementary aspects of this spiritual path. They strengthen and calm the mind and body. In this way they enable us to more easily follow the guidelines for right living.

The precepts of right living are relevant to expectant parents on two levels. First, the physical and emotional demands of pregnancy are sometimes unsettling to personal and family equilibrium. These guidelines can be simple reminders of basic priorities. Second, pregnancy is a preparation for parenthood. To be a parent is to be an example which will be impressed on your child's mind from birth—and before birth. These guidelines are reminders of the kind of model we can be for our children.

Restraints: Eliminating Negative Action

We place limits on ourselves in order to avoid the pitfalls of anger, violence, deceit, and greed. A basic premise of yoga is that we are essentially good. Therefore, if we eliminate negative behavior patterns, we emerge as purely loving human beings. As we are now, we are like diamonds in the rough. Once the dirt and grime are removed, the diamonds shine forth in their natural beauty. Once habits such as hurting, lying, stealing, and coveting are removed, our true nature emerges.

Baba Hari Dass, our teacher, was asked, "How can I learn to love?" His answer was simply: "Stop hating." When hate and its symptoms are removed, we become glittering diamonds, shining with love. The elimination of hate, hurting, lying, stealing, and hoarding is the purpose of practicing the yamas of yoga.

Noninjury

Noninjury means refraining from words, thoughts, and actions which cause physical or mental pain or harm to any living being, including ourselves. On the obvious level, it is synonymous with the First Commandment, "Thou shalt not kill." In yoga this demand extends beyond the human level into the animal kingdom. We are taught to refrain from killing animals (directly or indirectly) even for food. The usual yoga diet is vegetarian. The unnecessary taking of animal life is not considered consistent with spiritual life.

However, there are instances when the killing and eating of animals is tolerated even by yogis. In cold climates where the only food available is animal, as in Eskimo country or Tibetan mountain regions, the choice is made to preserve human rather than animal life. Also, when a person needs meat or fish for nutritional reasons, the choice is made in favor of the healthy preservation of the human being.

There is a third exception to the prohibition of killing that is relevant to pregnant women. In the fourth month of pregnancy, the spiritual heart of the baby becomes active. The mother's desires are now, to some extent, a reflection of the baby's needs in addition to her own. At this time if an expectant mother experiences a strong and persistent desire for flesh foods, the desire should be fulfilled. The meat or fish is needed for the child's development. The mother should sacrifice her nonviolent approach to diet for the healthy growth of her baby.

Noninjury extends far beyond dietetic stipulations. To not injure another living being requires control of anger and hate. On the gross level, noninjury demands that we refrain from all unkind acts and words. On a subtle level, it requires the elimination of all negative judgmental thoughts about ourselves and others. Freedom from harmful thoughts and actions is a demanding discipline. It requires patience and tolerance as we develop greater self-acceptance and acceptance of others.

During pregnancy, patience and tolerance of ourselves is especially essential. If we become judgmental of ourselves, our baby feels and absorbs the frustration we are reinforcing in ourselves. The most important thing to do when we become overcritical of ourselves is to relax and tune into that place inside ourselves where we feel whole and complete. Then acceptance is natural and our baby's environment positive.

Nonlying

There is one great deception in life: It is the illusion that each of us is a limited self trapped within the body, distinct from other beings and from God. We become slaves to this false, negative view of self, and the lies we tell serve to reinforce our sense of separateness. Think about it. We lie because we don't want someone to think badly of us—as if another's opinions could stain our true being. We lie in order to gain something for ourselves—money, success, self-importance. We do not believe that the honest expression of our true being—which is one with all other beings—is the way to satisfy every need.

By uncompromisingly not lying, we reinforce a positive self-image—the image of the self which is free. By practicing nonlying, we teach our children by example. We teach them even while they are in the womb that they can achieve self-worth and true success through total and honest self-expression.

Nonstealing

By not stealing we undermine two misconceptions about ourselves. The first misconception is the thought that we are not equal to others. Thus, for example, we feel less capable of paying than others, or we feel we are more deserving than others. We feel separate. In either case, we cannot steal if we recognize that all of us are equal manifestations of the same infinite power.

The second misconception at the root of stealing is doubt in our ability to care for ourselves. Therefore, we find it necessary to take what we have not earned. Yoga teaches us to have faith and to learn to accept the tides of emptiness or plenitude as they come to us.

Children are deeply influenced by an environment in which equality and faith are upheld. With these as their living example, they grow to realize their own potential as people who are loving and capable regardless of outer circumstances.

Noncollecting

Collecting, or hoarding, is the act of obtaining and keeping unnecessary things. The motivation for hoarding is like the second motivation mentioned for stealing: It is doubt. A basic insecurity lurking in the mind of the collector is the thought, "I might need this some day. What if I don't have it then?"

When we hold on to unnecessary things, it means we are worrying about the future instead of consciously being in the present. We do not trust that by living simply in the present we will learn to meet our needs satisfactorily in the future. Our minds are always filled with the words "What if . . . ?" "What if the price goes up? What if they stop carrying this brand? What if I run out?" So we collect. Collecting is not useful, intelligent planning. It is a wasteful activity grounded in fear.

To not collect in this culture, which encourages us to buy with enticing advertising everywhere, is a discipline in itself. It requires intelligence and foresight based on an understanding of our real needs. By placing reasonable limits on possessions, we become less obsessed with extraneous concerns because life becomes simpler. In this way, faith in our ability to meet the future becomes strong. We are able to discriminate between real and imagined needs.

The marketplace is filled with products designed to appeal to the collector mentality in parents. It would convince you that to have a healthy, happy baby you need disposable diapers, dressers full of baby clothes, a washer and dryer, a basinette, a changing table, a crib, a car bed, a cradle, a stroller and a carriage, a backpack and a cuddle seat and a high chair and a portable booster chair, and a jolly jumper, and a playpen, and two dozen bottles and a sterilizer, and canned formula, and anticolic medicines . . . the list is endless. You can become insecure thinking about all the money and space it will take to care for this infant. Raising a family, if one believes the advertisers, can seem like a nightmare!

Some products will no doubt make your life as a mother easier. If you can afford them, by all means buy them, but many other things will be useless. They will only clutter your house. All your baby really needs is a warm breast, enough diapers and clothes to last a few days before wash time, and a place to sleep.

Moderation in Sex

The power of sex to capture and imprison the mind, emotions, and senses is evidenced by the success of the advertising media in our consumer society. The mass idolization of sex is also reflected in the countless and ever-new ways it is vicariously presented in books, magazines, TV, and films. Sex, along with money and power, is accepted as one of the "ultimate" rewards in our restless and malcontent society.

Yoga philosophy is concerned with finding a middle path between indulgence and abstinence, and in the context of a loving relationship, sex is accepted as a natural and sacred expression of the love the couple shares. Overindulgence, whether it is expressed through physical overexertion, emotional anxiety, or mental preoccupation, prevents the experience of the transcendent state, which is the true expression of yoga.

Observances: Ways to Increase Positivity

The restraints, as we have discussed, are acts that should be avoided. The observances, on the other hand, are acts that should be performed to reinforce positivity.

The observances are based on the principle that as we think and act, so we tend to become. If we act lovingly, then we will become more loving. If we practice constraint, we will become more content. If we act in a spirit of surrender, then we will become more flexible human beings.

This type of "acting" is in no way insincere or phony; it is a practice. According to yoga, we are essentially good. Therefore, practicing good actions reinforces our true nature, the most sincere source of action. The conclusion naturally follows that all negative actions are, in a sense, "unreal" or phony. They cannot be considered real because they are based on delusion. All negative behavior is based on the misconception that we are separate rather than connected human beings.

Practicing cleanliness, contentment, self-discipline, right company, and surrender are ways to rid ourselves to a deluded identification with a negative self-image, and to gain a respect for our own true self-worth, as well as everyone else's.

Cleanliness

Cleanliness is physical hygiene and mental positivity. According to yoga, mind and body are interdependent and inseparable. The unhealthy body contributes to a troubled mind, and the healthy body facilitates a calm mind.

To be healthy, which is especially vital during pregnancy, the body must be kept externally and internally clean. Normal habits of cleanliness keep the external body clean. For maintaining a clean internal physical system, diet is of primary importance. Eating fresh and easily digested food is essential. Avoiding tobacco, alcohol, and drugs is always recommended but is especially stressed for pregnant women. These substances clog the system with toxins, and the effects are disturbing to your unborn child.

Many internal cleaning techniques are recommended in yoga, but most of these are not to be practiced by pregnant women. They are strenuous and can harm a child. Therefore, they will not be described.

Keeping the mind free of judgmental, cynical, and destructive thoughts is cleanliness of the mind. This mental cleanliness demands keeping careful watch over the activity of the mind. It is a difficult task which is aided by daily meditation.

Contentment

Contentment is a calm, accepting way of being. Fostering this state of mind requires that we act content. Acting content means that we foster mental, physical, and emotional stability in our lives.

Change for the sake of change does not create contentment. In this culture change is often equated with growth since our lives are lived at such a rapid pace. According to yoga philosophy, our spiritual progress is best served when we accept the demands of our life situation and meet the challenges we encounter with this acceptance.

During pregnancy, contentment is a state of mind especially to be desired, yet because of sensual sensitivities, emotional extremes, and the nesting tendency, it is sometimes hard to achieve. Therefore, it is important for expectant mothers to establish a way of acting content. Then contented action will begin to take root in the mind, and dissatisfactions and instabilities will be replaced by calm acceptance.

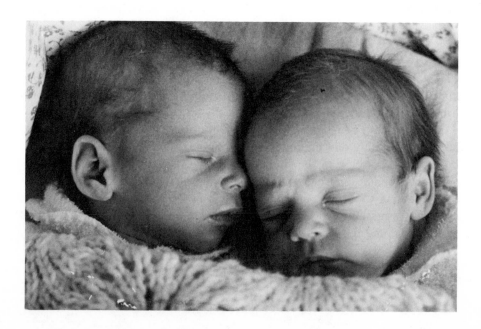

No matter how varied your day-to-day existence, certain planned activities can help to stabilize your life. Begin your day with a regular routine of yoga practice. It can be from thirty minutes to two hours. After eating breakfast, plan your day. Write down your five most important daily goals. Then put these into a timetable, or put them in order of priority from 1 to 5. By organizing our minds on paper, we can eliminate a great deal of frantic anxiety because we get a realistic view of the day's potential. Take ten minutes after lunch to recharge. Read an inspiring book or meditate. Before going to bed, review the day by writing down five ideas of importance to you. When you go to bed, pose to yourself a personal problem that needs solving. You may wake with an answer. Many people, including great scientists, have used this technique to gain original ideas.

By selecting three times of day—morning, noon, and evening—to turn within, you will become more content and better able to meet the inevitable physical and emotional changes that expectant parents face.

Self-discipline

Through disciplining one's way of life with yoga practices, the will power becomes strong. Yoga asserts that a strongly developed will is necessary for peace of mind.

Peace of mind is the ability to choose calmness rather than to be the victim of distracting and distressing thoughts. By choosing healthy, relaxing, and inspiring activities over laziness and overindulgence, we are disciplining our lives. In turn, our minds learn discipline from this regulation of our activities. The greatest need of a pregnant women is self-discipline. We need to control our tendencies toward laziness and indulgence throughout pregnancy, or we gain weight and lose our health. We need to control our fears and our breath throughout labor, or childbirth becomes a nightmare. The consequences of being undisciplined during pregnancy are so obvious that it is an opportune time to begin practicing yoga.

Right Company

The friends and books we choose make up our "company" according to this guideline. Choosing associations which are emotionally and mentally beneficial is a personal task that can sometimes be complex. It requires sincere self-searching.

The most comfortable company (whether in books or TV or people) can be

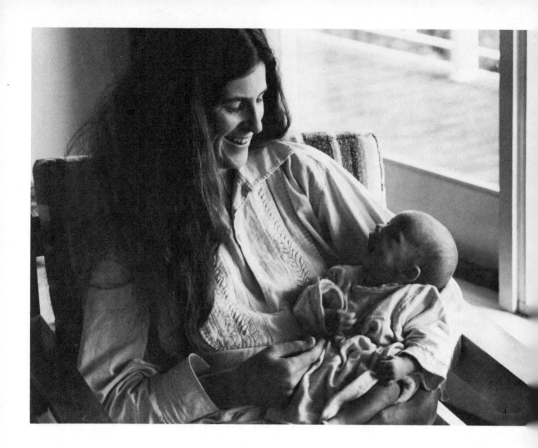

wasteful and even destructive, while a certain uneasiness in other relationships can be the impetus to growth. Or the opposite can be true. Comfortable
associations can bring self-affirmation, while tensions with others can be a
sign of incompatibility. Honesty and courage are demanded to determine
whether associations should be cultivated or discouraged.

As with every guideline for yogic living, the importance of right company
is heightened when you are pregnant. For example, you may reconsider as-
sociating with smokers. A simple habit such as this may require a boldness
you haven't expressed before. You may have to tell a smoking friend not to
smoke in your home. Being honest with your friend may be beneficial to the
growth of your friendship as well as to your child.

The emotional effects of your associations will begin to be felt by your
baby when you are four months pregnant—the time when the spiritual heart
becomes active. The baby is then affected by emotions and environment.
Reading uplifting literature, talking openly and honestly with friends, and
singing with others are associations which will have a positive effect on your
child.

Surrender

To practice surrender is to regard every circumstance as a blessing. It is to appreciate that both "good" and "bad" are equal opportunities for growth. Family life provides a multitude of opportunities to surrender. Therefore, it is a powerful vehicle for spiritual awakening.

There is nothing mystical or esoteric about surrender; it occurs in the mundane routines of life. Who'll do the dishes? What movie will we go to? Every question requiring compromise presents an opportunity to become a more spiritual human being—that is, a happier, healthier person.

Surrender always entails letting go of self-concern and replacing it with a concern for another. Parenthood teaches us to surrender self-concerns. The natural parental instincts of protection and self-sacrifice for the helpless being in our charge enables us to feel the immense gratification of total concern for another being.

4

BREATH:
THE SOURCE OF
VITALITY AND
RELAXATION

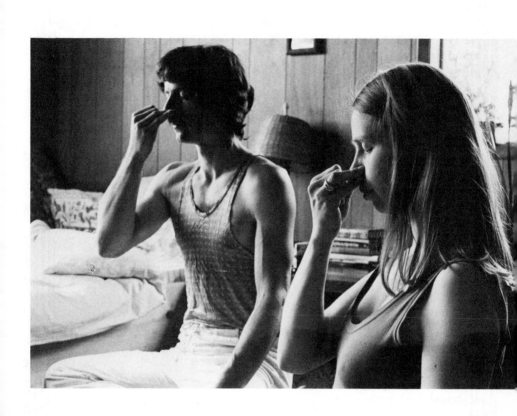

Breathing affects the whole system from the most subtle mental energy to the more gross, physical aspects of being. Breathing in a relaxed, natural manner throughout the day calms the mind and the body. In natural breathing, according to yoga, the abdomen extends slightly as air is inhaled and contracts as air is exhaled. To understand what we mean by natural breathing, put your hands on your abdomen. As you inhale, the abdomen will extend slightly; as you exhale, it will fall. This pattern of breathing should be cultivated during pregnancy. Breathing in a calming way will help to stabilize the emotions. It will give energy as each breath acts to renew the body. The positive effects of natural breathing will reach the baby in the womb.* The rhythmic in-and-out motions of your abdomen will be soothing to the baby.

The regular practice of breathing exercises can be used to great advantage during pregnancy. These exercises are very useful in giving a sense of tranquility. They contribute to the health of the body by clearing it of excess mucus, soothing the nerves, aiding digestion, relieving constipation, strengthening the sexual glands, assisting circulation, and combatting fatigue.

The effect of breathing exercises is quite subtle though very strong. For the greatest benefit, practice these exercises daily. A routine will take fifteen to twenty minutes. The most effective way to practice breathing exercises is to begin a routine of yoga practice with them first thing in the morning. It is helpful to make a habit of doing them at the same time every day.

There are six exercises included here. The four purification breathing techniques are usually done in the order suggested here. Alternate Nostril Breathing, Skull Shining, and Anal Sphincter Contraction will be beneficial to everyone throughout pregnancy. However, please note that Fire Cleansing should be stopped at the end of the fourth month and resumed again only after the birth.

One of the other two exercises described will be particularly helpful to women who live in a cold climate or feel cold. The other will be useful in a hot climate or when the body feels too hot. These exercises have additional benefits which are mentioned in the following descriptions of each. Read them and practice them. Then you can establish the best routine for your own needs.

A few words of caution. The breathing techniques we have presented here are extremely gentle and soothing and involve little or no breath retention.

*For a detailed discussion of the fetal environment, see *In the Beginning: Your Baby's Brain before Birth* listed under Suggested Readings, page 148.

We have taught these exercises to hundreds of men and women over the past ten years and not a single person has complained of dizziness. However, it is quite difficult to do breathing exercises correctly with a book's guidance alone. Be aware of how these exercises are affecting you. If you feel discomfort, discontinue them. We sincerely believe you will have no difficulty with any of the breathing exercises we describe here, but only you can be the judge of your body's reactions.

Cleaning the Nasal Passages

This is a very simple, yet highly effective method for cleaning the nasal passages of mucus and accumulated dirt. We recommend that this cleansing technique be done every morning just before practicing the breathing techniques that follow.

Fill a plastic watering can with lukewarm water. Place one teaspoon of sea salt in the watering can and stir until it has dissolved in the water. Now ascertain which of your two nostrils is more "open" than the other and insert the spout of the watering can into that nostril. Tilt your head to the side and, breathing through your mouth, begin to pour the salted water into your nostril. The water will automatically run from one nostril through to the other. After a few seconds remove the spout from that nostril, turn your head in the opposite direction, and repeat the process. This is an absolutely safe procedure which we have even shared with young children.

The Four Purification Techniques

1. Alternate Nostril Breathing

This exercise is designed to purify and balance the nervous system and allow prana (life-force energy) to flow freely through the body. It helps the mind to become still and clear. It should be practiced through the entire pregnancy.

METHOD

1 Sit in any comfortable cross-legged position.
2 Put the thumb of the right hand on the right nostril and the last two fingers of the right hand on the left nostril. Open the left nostril and gently exhale all the air out of that side while closing the right nostril with the thumb.

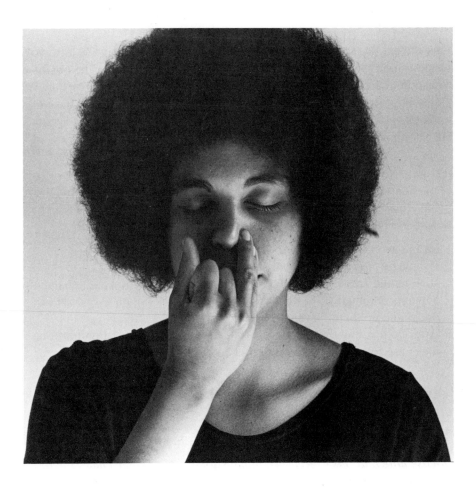

3 Slowly breathe in through the left nostril until the lungs are full, making as
  little sound as possible. When breathing in, allow the diaphragm to rise
  upward slowly, and keep the abdomen relaxed.
4 After the breath is completed, close the left nostril, lift the right thumb,
  and slowly exhale through the right nostril.
5 Without a pause, inhale through the right nostril as in step 3, and exhale
  through the left nostril as in step 4.

This is one round. Start with 10 rounds and gradually increase to 25
rounds.

2. Skull Shining

This is a gentle, shallow breathing exercise specifically designed to remove congestion in the nasal and bronchial areas. It also stimulates the organs of digestion and elimination, rids the body of excess carbon dioxide, and replenishes it with an abundant supply of oxygen; it invigorates the entire nervous system. This exercise should be done through the entire pregnancy, but very gently.

METHOD

Skull shining consists of a series of rhythmic rapid shallow breathing movements done from the naval area. Gentle effort is applied only to the exhalation; the inhalation is passive.

1 Sit in any comfortable cross-legged position.
2 Exhale by pushing the abdomen inward with a gentle pistonlike stroke. As soon as the stroke is completed, the abdomen is relaxed and inhalation happens automatically. Repeat at the rate of one breath every few seconds, and do 20 to 50 repetitions.
3 After completing the repetitions, take a long, slow inhalation until the lungs are filled and concentrate between and behind the eyebrows for a few seconds. Then exhale slowly.

One round of 20 to 50 repetitions is sufficient during pregnancy.

3. Fire Cleansing

(Please note that this exercise should be done only until the end of the fourth month of pregnancy.)

Fire cleansing is designed to stimulate and strengthen the glands and organs that are responsible for digestion and assimilation. Growth, strength, and resistance to disease depend on the proper functioning of these organs. Done regularly and correctly, Fire Cleansing eliminates impurities in the abdominal area; it aids and strengthens the digestive fires by increasing and controlling the special life force necessary for digestion and assimilation. Also, it tones the entire abdominal area, making it fit for childbearing.

METHOD

1 You can practice this exercise standing with the legs spread about a foot apart, knees slightly bent, and hands on the thighs, fingers turned inward.

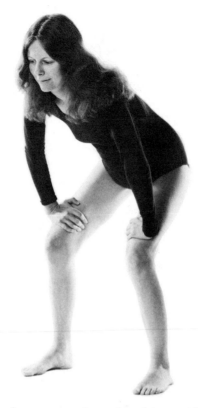

Or you can do it sitting in any cross-legged position, with the hands on the knees, fingers turned inward.

2 Either way, just exhale all the air from the lungs and lower the chin to the chest, if possible.

3 With the breath held out, vigorously pull the abdomen inward so that the navel is drawn towards the spine. Relax the abdomen and allow it to return to its normal position. Rapidly repeat this movement 20 to 40 times on a single-expelled breath.

4 When it comes time to take another breath, stop pulling on the abdomen and breathe in slowly. This completes one round. Do one or two rounds of 20 to 40 pulls.

4. Anal Sphincter Contraction

This exercise stimulates the energy center at the base of the spine and pushes prana to all parts of the body. It is also helpful in relieving hemorrhoids and constipation.

This exercise is extremely important during pregnancy because it strengthens the sexual organs and glands. Moreover, it strengthens the power of the downward-pushing energy called apana vayu, whose function it is to push the baby out of the birth canal. This exercise should be practiced regularly during the pregnancy and should also be continued after the birth as it will bring the sexual organs back into shape very quickly.

METHOD

1 Sit in any comfortable cross-legged position (the Shakti pose is best during pregnancy; see page 84).
2 Inhale slowly and retain the breath. Turn the chin down into the chest.
3 Then, while holding the breath, contract and relax the anus in quick succession. Do 20 to 50 contractions on a single inhaled breath.
4 When it comes time to exhale, lift the chin slowly and breathe out gently. Do up to two rounds of 20 to 50 contractions at one sitting.

Additional Breathing Techniques

1. Piercing the Sun

This exercise is designed to increase the heat in the body and therefore should be practiced only when you feel cold or when the weather is cold. In addition to increasing body temperature, this exercise increases digestive strength. It can be done at any stage of pregnancy.

METHOD

1 Sit in any comfortable cross-legged position.
2 Inhale gently through the right nostril, while keeping the left nostril closed with the fingers as for Alternate Nostril Breathing. Then, when the inhalation is complete, close the right nostril and gently exhale through the left nostril.
3 When the exhalation is complete, once again inhale through the right nostril and exhale through the left. Continue this for 12 to 25 inhalations at one sitting.

2. The Cooling Breath

This exercise is designed to cool the system and is very useful when your body temperature is high or when the weather is extremely warm. If practiced regularly, it cools overheated organs and corrects bile disorders. It is also very useful in alleviating false hunger and thirst, and it purifies the system of toxins. It should not be practiced in the winter or when the body is too cold.

METHOD

1 Sit in any comfortable cross-legged position.
2 Roll the tongue lengthwise and protrude it a little from the lips.
3 Inhale fully through this "tube," and then exhale through both nostrils, without retaining the breath.
4 Repeat this practice 25 to 30 times.

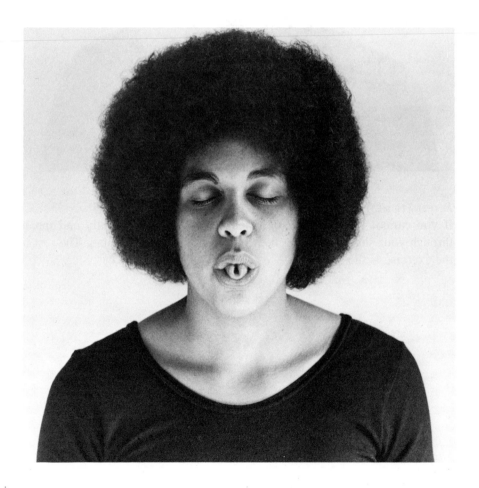

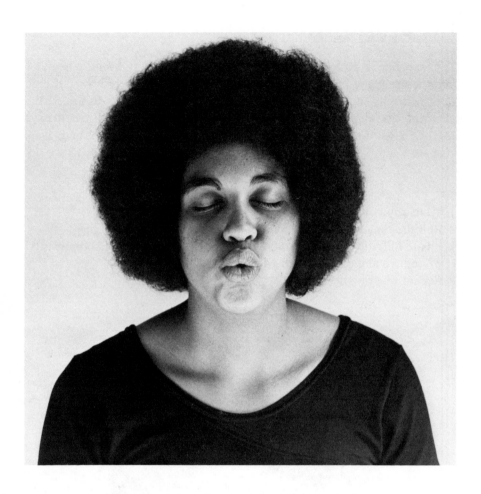

ALTERNATE METHOD

If you cannot roll your tongue, then purse your lips slightly and inhale through your slightly opened mouth, with a light hissing sound. The rest of the exercise is the same.

5

MEDITATION: FREEING THE MIND

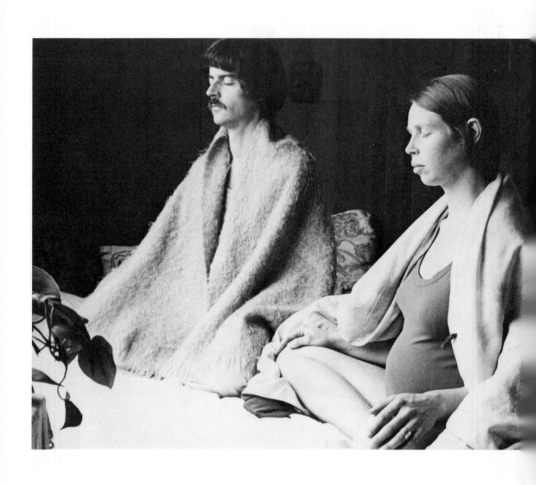

Meditation can be defined as freeing the mind from undesirable thoughts. The process of getting rid of negative thinking is essential to peace, to happiness, to love, and to health. Of course, it is not easy to change mental habits that have been with us all of our lives. But if we want to enjoy peace of mind, the mind's position as ruler must be usurped and the ruler made slave. This can't be done in a day, a week, or even a year. Meditation is a long and vigilant practice that gradually creates a new awareness and sensitivity. True mediation is a lifetime endeavor—but this shouldn't put anyone off; after all, if we really value peace of mind, we will be willing to make efforts to attain it.

During pregnancy, creating a beautiful world through beautiful thoughts is especially important and wonderful. It is important because your thoughts affect your baby. It's wonderful because when your baby feels the emotions generated by positive thoughts, you experience a double happiness. When a pattern of positivity affects the mind, then everything is seen as perfect. We see the good side of everything. We learn to be happier and more loving during every daily experience. When we're in this state of mind, nothing can go wrong. As St. Paul said, "Everything works for good for those who love God."

Meditation can help clear the mind of undesired thoughts. There are many meditation techniques prescribed by teachers according to their particular backgrounds. Some of these methods are appropriate for one person but not for another. As our own teacher, Baba Hari Dass, points out, "One medicine cannot cure all diseases." We'd like to share a few possible meditations with you. Experiment with each until you find the one or two which help clear your mind and create a sense of peace.

Meditation should be practiced daily. The light of a single match can be blown out quickly. But if more twigs and branches are added to it, the wind can't hurt it. It's true with your mind also. One short period of meditation can't overcome all your negativity. But regular meditation will make your positive mind strong. The analogy can be taken further. Timing is important in building a fire. If you put a huge log on top of your match it will go out. Similarly, if you force yourself to meditate for too long a period of time, your mind will rebel and nothing will be accomplished. Ten minutes a day of positive concentration are better than two hours of daydreaming. On the other hand, if you forget to add fuel to your fire, it will die out. Likewise, if you meditate sporadically, the positivity of your meditation will lose momentum.

Mantra Meditation

Aditya hridayum punyam sarv shatru bena shenam.
All evil vanishes from him who keeps the sun in his heart.

This statement is a mantra—a spiritually powerful statement, word, or thought which is repeated over and over and over again. A few years ago, using this particular mantra was a ritual at Lama Foundation, a spiritual community in New Mexico. The fifteen or so adults living there would wake at 5:00 A.M. We would silently make our way to the meditation hall. Then we would rhythmically repeat this mantra in Sanskrit for approximately one hour. This experience taught me the positive power of mantra meditation. After meditating with the mantra, all my tensions, anxieties, and doubts were relieved, and I felt loving.

A mantra has a special meaning for the person meditating with it. Often the words are in an ancient language like Sanskirt, Tibetan, Greek, Hebrew, or Arabic, depending on the religion they originated from. These old languages originated in a time when religion and nature were better integrated into the daily experience of people. Therefore, it is believed that the sounds of these languages have a finer, more natural vibration. The words have a greater physical and emotional effect because they are closely tuned to the subtle workings of the body and mind.

However, mantras in modern languages are also often helpful. The familiarity of meaning can help you absorb the positive thoughts embodied in the words. As the mind dwells more and more on uplifting thoughts, the whole personality becomes an expression of love and joy.

Whether repeated aloud or silently, in an ancient language or in English, the mantra has a transforming effect. As the meditator focuses attention on the sound of the mantra, the habitual wanderings of the mind—which are at best useless and at worst destructive—are gradually stilled, leaving the mind free to receive inspiration. The repeated use of a mantra gives it the power to penetrate the subconscious mind, dissolving the deep-seated fears and doubts which cause anger, jealousy, hate, and insecurity and allowing love and faith to emerge.

To practice mantra meditation formally, sit on the floor in a comfortable cross-legged position with your spine straight. If sitting on the floor is difficult, use a chair, but keep the spine erect. Close your eyes, and let the tensions go out of your mind and body.

Now repeat your chosen mantra over and over and over again to yourself. Let your being absorb the meaning of the words. Don't analyze them. Just understand them through feeling them. For example, feel as though they are washing your body with a light that penetrates inside you and radiates out beyond you. Do this for fifteen concentrated minutes. Then slowly stretch and move.

Breath and Mantra

Mantras are often coordinated with the breath. To do this, feel as though you are inhaling the words into your abdomen as you breathe in. Feel as though you are exhaling the words as you breathe out. You may find it beneficial to take this "breathing" of your mantra one step further. As you inhale, feel that the words are reaching into your being. They are touching your heart and reaching into your abdomen. As you exhale, feel the words to be reaching out to the extremities of your body. Feel that with each breath your mantra is vitalizing your whole being. Or you may wish to feel the inhalation affecting your whole body, while the exhalation sends the mantra out into the world, spreading a feeling of bliss all around you.

Hum Sah Meditation

One meditation technique which coordinates breath and mantra repetition is the Hum Sah meditation. It is a calming yet energizing exercise. Sit as you would for any other meditation. Close your eyes. Breathe deeply and evenly several times. Allow the mind to be calm and the emotions to settle. Now focus on the baby inside and begin to watch the movement of your breath. As you inhale imagine that you hear the sound "hum." As you exhale imagine the sound "sah." This meditation can be done for ten to fifteen minutes in the beginning. It can be increased if you desire.

Mantra through the Day

Mantra can be maintained throughout the day's activities. You can repeat a mantra as you do dishes or cook. When the mantra becomes deeply seated in your subconscious you will find it is being repeated even while you are involved in your work or when reading or talking. Perhaps mantra meditation is so powerful because it can be carried with you throughout the day.

Mantra for Pregnancy

There is a mantra recommended for use during pregnancy. It is:

> Dear God I take trust in you.
> Bless me with a healthy baby.

This mantra is repeated before going to bed so that as you sleep your subconscious mind will be filled with devotion and gratitude to God for the blessing of bearing a child. Thus your sleep will be positively affected.

The mantra for pregnancy is also recommended for labor. With the mind dwelling on God and on the blessing you are about to receive, you can experience bliss despite the pain of childbirth.

Ram Meditation

The heart is the focus of many forms of meditation. Having a soft and open spiritual heart is one aim of all meditations. For someone who is becoming a mother, a warm, soft, and open heart is needed to meet the challenges of childbirth and child rearing. Children need this heart space in a mother. In yoga, the mantra "Ram" is the traditional mantra of the heart.

To practice this mantra, sit as always recommended with the back straight. Close your eyes. Focus on your breath. Take a few deep, slow breaths into your abdomen. Feel the relaxation this breathing brings to you. Imagine a flame eight-finger-breadths wide in the center of your chest. Feel that the flame is melting away all hardness of your heart. As you visualize this flame, repeat the mantra, "Ram, Ram, Ram" silently over and over for approximately fifteen minutes.

Tratak: Candle Gazing Meditation

Tratak, or candle gazing, is both a meditation and a cleansing exercise. Simply stated, tratak is staring at an object (often a candle) without blinking. This visual concentration directs the mind through the aid of the sense of sight. As you stare in this concentrated manner, the mind focuses on one object and extraneous thoughts subside. Calmness of mind and increased will power are the result of practicing tratak regularly.

Tratak is also considered a cleansing exercise in yoga. Cleansing exercises are practices which clean or purify the body. They remove disease caused by excess mucus and deranged bile. A balanced amount of mucus and bile are necessary to the healthy functioning of the body. When these substances are present in excess or become deranged, however, the body discharges them through disease. Although most of the cleansing exercises practiced in yoga are not recommended for pregnant women, tratak is a safe and beneficial purification method for them.

When you first practice tratak, the eyes water and the mucus in the nasal area is loosened. Practiced daily, tratak can prevent colds, sinus problems, and headaches caused by blockage in the sinus areas. As stated, it is also excellent for developing concentration and will power, two qualities essential for successful childbirth.

To practice tratak, place a candle at the level of the eyes, about an arm's length from you. Sit comfortably in a meditation position with your spine straight. Stare at the flame without blinking. Begin by practicing for three to five minutes and work your way up to fifteen minutes, unless you have problems with your vision or are either near- or far-sighted. If you do have visual problems, do tratak for only three minutes. After the time is up, close your eyes and concentrate on the afterimage of the flame. You may continue the exercise for a prolonged period by alternating between concentrating on the flame (eyes open) and concentrating on the afterimage (eyes closed), giving a few minutes to each.

6

PHYSICAL POSTURES: ASANAS FOR PREGNANCY

The complexities of a technological society are such that it is difficult to remember that we, like the animal kingdom, are a part of nature. Our life styles divorce us almost completely from any instinctual heritage. We ride in cars rather than walk; our food comes from supermarket shelves rather than directly from the earth. Nature, in almost every way, seems far removed from our daily existence.

Pregnancy reminds us of our unity with all of nature. It allows us the opportunity to know undeniably that we share the instinctual desire of all animals to preserve their species. We feel that our life serves as a vehicle for new life.

If our way of life enabled us to observe animals in their natural environment, we could learn a great deal about our own instinctual needs and natural inclinations during pregnancy. I've noticed, for example, that our cats have sought more quietness, affection, and rest while pregnant. They have also tended to stay closer to home during the entire gestation. These patterns can be seen as well in the natural needs of women for security, peace, and love during pregnancy.

Ancient yogis, who were master observers of animal life, recognized that many human needs and ailments could be fulfilled or cured by intelligent application of what they learned from their observations. This practice of observing animals is the source of the yogic system of physical postures or asanas. These ancient yogis withdrew from civilization in order to meditate in solitude. Living in the jungle, they became attuned to the ways of nature. They paid particular attention to animals, fish, birds, and insects. They noticed that these animals instinctively reacted to illness or distress by assuming certain bodily positions which served to provide relief. They then experimented on themselves with these postures and found that many were beneficial to the human system as well. Through continued experimentation they developed a system of physical postures that, when properly and regularly practiced, provide glowing health, strength, and stamina. Of the thousands of postures discovered, eighty-four were considered to be the main postures. Of these eighty-four main postures, twenty-five postures are presented here for their particular benefit to pregnant women.

Suggestions for Maximum Benefit

During pregnancy, when your emotions may become unsteady, grounding yourself with regular, concentrated, but gentle physical exercise will aid your equilibrium. Also, many of us get tired during gestation. Yoga asanas energize the body. This vitalizing effect aids the development of your baby as well. When your body is regularly recharged throughout pregnancy, then your energy will naturally be strong for labor. The asanas we present for pregnancy are aimed at the body parts which need special strength and flexibility for childbearing. These asanas also activate a subtle energy called apana vayu which helps push the child steadily downward during labor.

Some asanas can be dangerous if practiced during pregnancy. *No inverted poses should be performed after the fourth month.* Others are dangerous if practiced beyond the time we have indicated in this book. The asanas we recommend are perfectly safe for the periods specified. When there is any chance of a detrimental effect, we recommend the asana be discontinued for the remainder of your pregnancy. If you have health problems such as a weak back, or if discomfort arises while practicing the asanas, it may be wise to consult your physician. After the *second month* of pregnancy particular care should be exercised when practicing any postures that involve back bending. In the program recommended here, this would include Sun Salutation, Half-Locust, Alligator, Bow, Cobra, Camel, and Fish.

It is not necessary to do all the asanas illustrated. Do them according to your ability, strength, and time. Do not be rigid about your routine. Make asanas a daily habit, but if discomfort arises from a particular exercise, rest. If it feels necessary, discontinue that asana. If you are stiff and an asana is difficult, do it to the best of your ability. Practice slowly and gently. Patiently go a little further each day. Gradually you will be amazed by the increase in flexibility and strength. "Do not force" is the cardinal rule of yoga. You are trying to relax your body. Force will constrict it and possibly damage it.

If you feel tired, stop and rest for a brief time. Lie down on your back or stomach and breathe deeply and slowly into your abdomen. Feel the breath gently relax your whole body. Frequent short stops will help you to keep in touch with the effect each asana has on you. The only danger is that the mind may wander and your calm will be lost. Approach each short rest as a meditation, a time to still the mind by concentrating on the breath.

The breath is important throughout your asana routine. It should always be slow and smooth. When you inhale, the abdomen should extend slightly as the air reaches the bottom of the lungs. When you exhale, it should contract slightly as the air is emptied from the lungs. Because the movement of air is visible in the movement of the abdomen, it is said that natural breathing (according to yoga) is breathing through the nostrils into the abdomen. Unless otherwise stated, breathe "naturally" during all asanas. Your body movement during asanas should be harmonized with your breath. You should feel that your breath is moving your body in and out of each position. Generally the breath is slowly exhaled as you bend forward and inhaled as you bend back. In a standing position, exhale bending the head down, inhale coming back into an erect position. There are very few exceptions to these general guidelines to breathing for asanas.

You should practice asanas on an empty stomach. Slow, rhythmic exercise is a good way to begin the day. But if morning is an inconvenient time, then be sure it's been at least two hours after eating when you begin to exercise.

Do not do yoga exercises while the body is cold. During pregnancy frequent baths are enjoyable. A bath may be taken before asanas. The warmth of the water will make your body more flexible, and the routine will be more satisfying.

Begin your asanas with a warmup period. The hands can be briskly rubbed together to create warmth. Then the whole body can be energetically rubbed. Begin at your feet, and work up your body—lower legs, knees, thighs, stomach, buttocks, chest, back, neck, arms, face, and head. After that brief body rub, jump up and down moving your legs and arms for a few minutes. Then swing your arms, stretch your back, dance a bit. Now you are ready to begin.

Asanas should not be done for six weeks after your baby is born. Then begin to practice them again. Begin slowly and gradually. Increase the number and difficulty of the exercises gradually. If yoga is done throughout pregnancy the body will assume its previous shape within a week after giving birth. The skin will have no stretch marks and the belly will be firm. With the help of a postnatal program the internal organs will be healed and the system quickly returned to normal.

Asanas are primarily concerned with positively affecting the life-force energy, or prana, in the human system. According to yoga theory, properly functioning prana is responsible for physical, emotional, and mental well-being, while derangement of this energy is held to be the cause of physical ailments, emotional imbalance, and mental dullness. Asanas powerfully affect the flow of prana in the system, and one gradually becomes more sensitive to this flow after some practice. Signs of awakened life-force energy are feelings of mental clarity, emotional harmony, and physical energy.

We recommend that you do the following asanas with care at the end of the *fourth* and *seventh* months to adjust your practice to the new stage of pregnancy reached. While it is desirable to do as many asanas as possible that pertain to one's stage on a daily basis, this will necessarily be different from woman to woman, according to each one's health and the time she has available. However, there is no question that if a mother-to-be is consistent in practicing asanas regularly, her health, vitality, and stamina will be greatly improved.

ASANAS TO BE DISCONTINUED'AT END OF FOURTH MONTH

1 Sun Salutation
2 Shoulder Stand
3 Half-Locust
4 Alligator
5 The Bow
6 Cobra

ASANAS TO BE DISCONTINUED AT END OF SEVENTH MONTH

7 Raised Lotus
8 Hidden Lotus
9 Half-Spinal Twist
10 Wind-Releasing Pose
11 Stretched Bow
12 Camel

ASANAS THAT MAY BE DONE THROUGH ENTIRE PREGNANCY

13 Fish
14 Shakti
15 Tadpole
16 Star
17 Cowhead
18 Nobleman Pose
19 Lying Nobleman Pose
20 Cat
21 Standing Triangle Pose
22 Palm Tree
23 Tree
24 Standing Splits
25 Corpse

The Asanas

1. Sun Salutation

This asana is actually a series of eleven flowing movements and postures, each connected to the other in a definite sequence. Traditionally the Sun Salutation is done as a way of greeting the new day when the sun comes up in the morning. For our purposes it is best done at this time, although it is beneficial at any time.

METHOD:

1 Assume the posture shown in the photograph. Make sure feet are neatly together, spine straight, posture erect but not stiff. Breathe normally.
2 *Inhale* while bending backward.
3 *Exhale*, bringing the head as close to the knees as possible while keeping the legs straight.

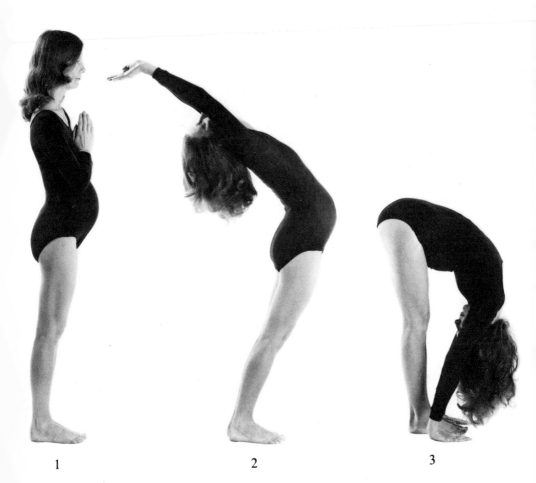

1   2   3

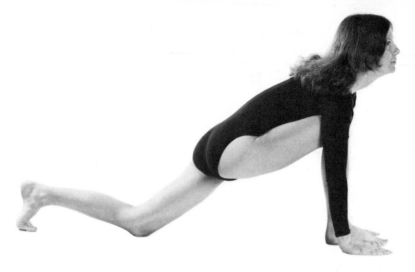

4 *Inhale,* stretching the left leg back and resting the left knee on the floor. Keeping the hands on the floor, stretch the head and upper body upward.

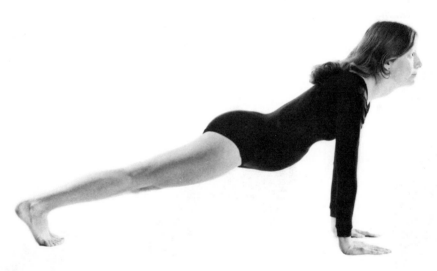

5 Stretch the right leg back, and while briefly *holding the breath,* hold the body erect.

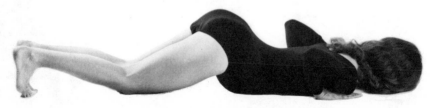

6 *Exhale,* touching the knees, chest, and forehead to the floor.

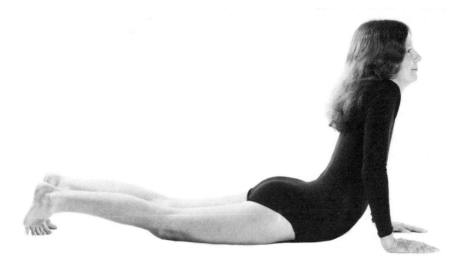

7 *Inhale,* stretching the upper body upward as far as possible. Keep the arms straight, keep the head erect (do not bend it back), and allow the shoulders to hunch up.

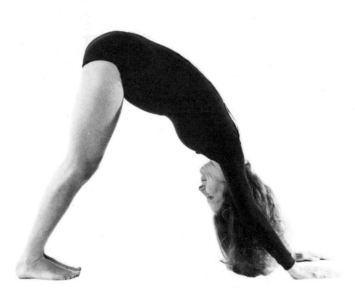

8 *Exhale,* straightening the legs, body, and arms, and bending at the waist.

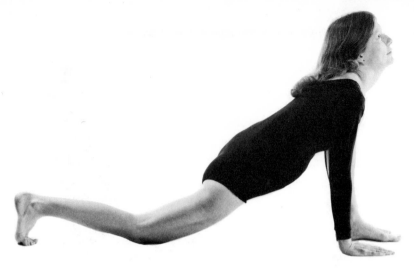

9 *Inhale* exactly as in step 4, only this time with the right leg back and the left leg forward.

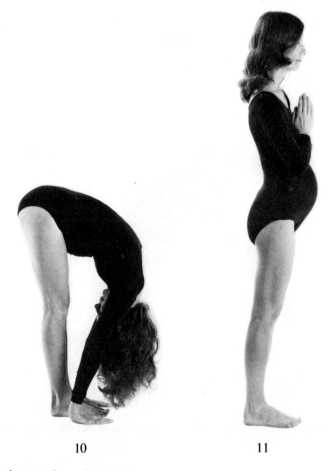

10   11

10 *Exhale* exactly as in step 3.
11 Resume posture as in step 1.

The Sun Salutation can be done several times, according to strength and ability. Eventually a graceful and flowing style of movement will emerge.

TIME PERIOD: Can be done until the end of the fourth month.

BENEFITS: This asana contains many other asanas in its movement and thus has many benefits. Among other effects, it increases general vitality, improves digestion, keeps the body trim and supple, and develops concentration and gracefulness.

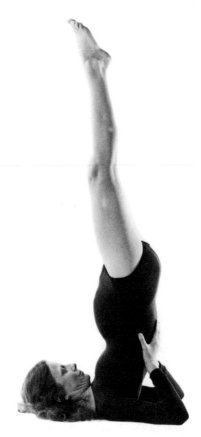

2. Shoulder Stand

METHOD: Inhale slowly while raising the legs. Try to straighten the spine as much as possible. Support the back with your hands as in the photograph. Hold the position for 1 to 5 minutes, closing the eyes and concentrating on the throat region. Breathe naturally while in the position. Exhale as you bring your legs down when you come out of the position.

TIME PERIOD: Can be done until the end of the fourth month.

BENEFITS: The name for this asana in Sanskrit is Sarvang, which means "whole body"; this is in apparent recognition of the effect on the whole body of this wonderful asana. It works on the thyroid and parathyroid glands in the neck, squeezing the blood out of these glands. Regular practice of this asana aids metabolism, growth, and nutrition and corrects body structure; it also promotes the health of the circulatory, respiratory, alimentary, genitourinary, and nervous systems. In addition, it supplies large quantities of blood to the spinal roots of the nerves. It is helpful in urinary disorders and female organ and menstrual difficulties. Small wonder it is called the mother of the asanas!

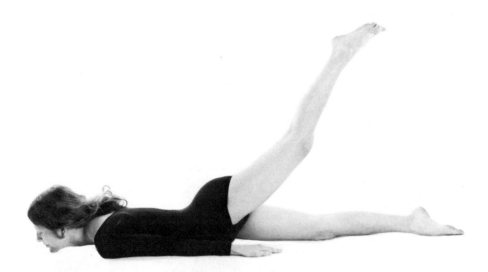

3. Half-Locust

METHOD: Lie on the floor, chest and stomach downward. Place the chin on the floor, hands underneath the body. Using the arms and hands (palms toward the floor) as a support, inhale while raising the legs as in the photograph. Breathe normally while holding that position for between 15 and 30 seconds, then exhale *gently* as you bring your legs back to their normal position. Repeat according to strength once or twice more.

TIME PERIOD: Can be done until the end of the fourth month.

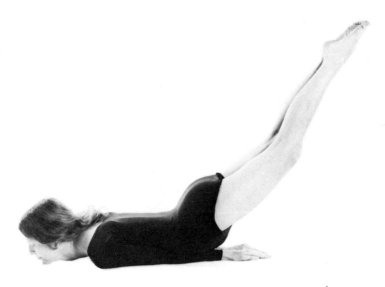

BENEFITS: Tones the spinal column, develops elasticity, prevents pain in the lumbar and sacral regions, relieves constipation, increases appetite, tones the ovaries and uterus, and reduces fat.

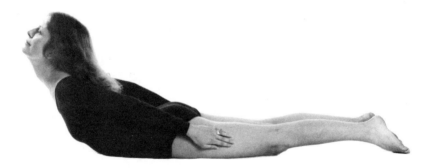

4. Alligator

METHOD: Lie on the floor facing down, hands at the sides. Keeping the legs on the floor, raise the upper body without support of the arms. Inhale, raising the body, breathe normally in position, and exhale, lowering the body.

TIME PERIOD: Can be done until the end of the fourth month.

BENEFITS: Same as for Half-Locust pose. Also strengthens the back muscles.

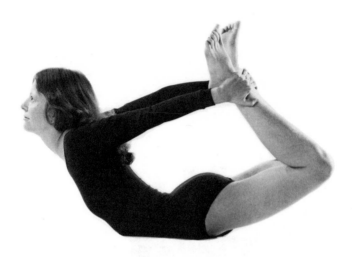

5. The Bow

METHOD: Lie on the stomach. Inhaling, grasp the right ankle with the right hand, and the left ankle with the left hand. Gently but firmly, pull the thighs off the floor. Now begin to rock back and forth gently on the entire abdominal area, holding the breath. Maintain this rocking motion for approximately 10 to 20 seconds. Exhale *gently* and rest in the Corpse pose.

TIME PERIOD: Should be stopped at the end of the fourth month.

BENEFITS: Reduces fat. Tones the spinal column and makes it more elastic. Helps to alleviate gastrointestinal disorders. Develops appetite. Also helps to tone the female organs.

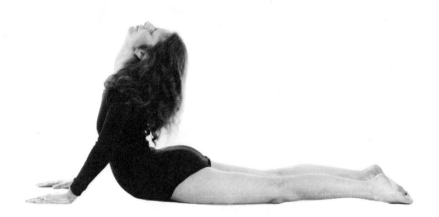

6. Cobra

METHOD: Lie face-down on the floor. Place the hands with palms down on the floor, underneath the shoulders and next to the chest. Raise the chest and head off the floor as far as possible, arching the neck backward, inhaling as you arch upward. Breathe in the arched position for a few seconds, then exhale and reverse the arch, easing the body gently back to the floor. Do the asana two or three times. NOTE: If any discomfort is felt from pressure on the abdomen, it is advisable to stop this asana until after the baby is born.

TIME PERIOD: Can be done until the end of the fourth month, depending on comfort.

BENEFITS: Brings energy to the sixth chakra, the mental center, seated in the forehead. Stretches and stimulates the spine and the blood circulation and exercises and strengthens the pineal, pituitary, adrenal, and thyroid glands. Also strengthens the back.

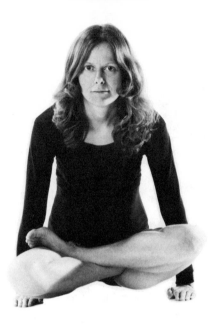

7. Raised Lotus

METHOD: Sit with legs straight ahead. Place the left foot on the right thigh. Then place the right foot on the left thigh. This is the Lotus pose. Place the palms on the floor and inhale, raising the whole body off the floor, supported only on the hands. Breathe normally in this position. Exhale when returning the body to the floor. NOTE: This is an advanced asana and should not be forced.

TIME PERIOD: Can be practiced until the end of the seventh month.

BENEFITS: Brings elasticity to the hips, knees, and foot joints; strengthens the wrists, hands, and abdominal walls. NOTE: The Lotus is the best pose for meditation. The heart does not have to pump much blood into the legs; the position of the crossed legs and the erect back facilitates an alert and attentive mind.

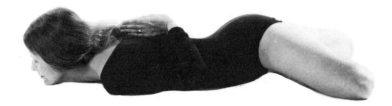

8. Hidden Lotus

METHOD: Take the Lotus pose as described in the Raised Lotus above. Now come to a "standing" position on the knees, then lean forward and allow the hips to swivel. Fold your hands together in the prayer position and hold them in this position. Breathe naturally and maintain the pose for 20 to 30 seconds.

TIME PERIOD: Can be done until the end of the seventh month.

BENEFITS: Stretches the upper back and shoulders, the groin area, and the lower stomach and has a toning effect on the entire system.

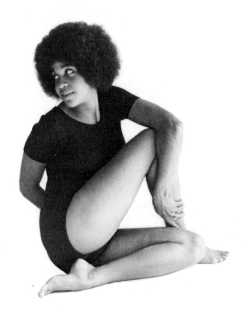

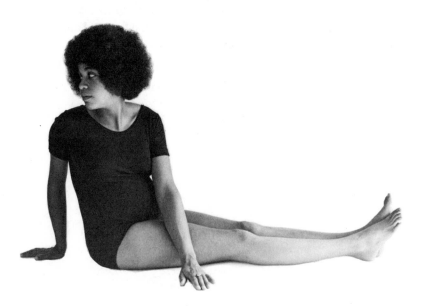

9. Half-Spinal Twist

There are two variations, which can be done according to ability. Spinal twists should always be done in both directions.

METHOD: Sit with the left heel pressing the sitting bone. Raise the right leg, cross the foot over the folded left leg, and place the right foot on the floor at about the middle of the left thigh. Twist the spine to the right. Bring the left hand around to the inside of the bent right knee and grasp the lower left leg (ankle, if possible). Put the right arm behind the back, turning the head and looking over the right shoulder as far as possible. Repeat on the other side. Breathe slowly and deeply while in the pose.

ALTERNATE METHOD: Sit with the legs stretched out in front of you, then extend both arms to the right side as in the picture. Stretch gently. Then do the same on the left side. There should be no strain whatsoever. Breathe easily and gently.

TIME PERIOD: Can be done until the end of the seventh month.

BENEFITS: Increases blood supply to the nervous system and stretches the back in an unusual manner, thus relieving various muscular tensions.

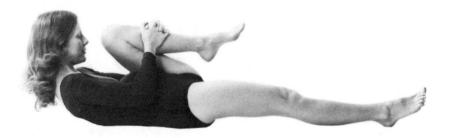

10. Wind-Releasing Pose, I and II

METHODS: For method I, lie on the back and inhale, bending one leg and pulling it toward the chest, while simultaneously bringing the head and neck as close to the knee as possible. Hold the breath in this position for a few seconds, then exhale while returning to the lying position. Repeat with the other leg. For method II, follow the same instructions, but raise both legs together.

TIME PERIOD: Can be done until the end of the seventh month.

BENEFITS: Both methods push poisonous gases out of the abdomen. They help cure indigestion, acidity, flatulence, and constipation. They also help tone the gastric glands and invigorate abdominal nerves and muscles.

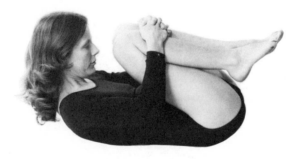

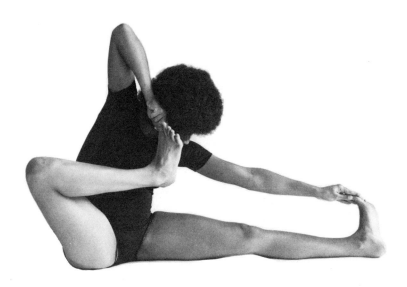

11. Stretched Bow, I and II

METHODS: For Stretched Bow I, sit with the legs forward. Take hold of the right toe with the left hand and pull the foot up to the left ear. At the same time, touch the left toe with the right hand (the left leg remains stretched forward on the floor). Hold the position for 10 to 20 seconds, breathing deeply and slowly. Then do the same on the other side. Breathe naturally, without strain.

For Stretched Bow II, sit with the legs stretched forward. Take hold of the right toe with the right hand and pull it up to the right ear. Meanwhile, take hold of the left toe with the left hand. Then do the same on the other side. Breathe naturally, without strain.

TIME PERIOD: Can be done until the end of the seventh month.

BENEFITS: Stretches the internal hip area and the legs; strengthens the arms and the back.

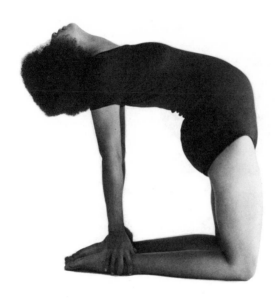

12. Camel

METHOD: Kneel on both knees, with the legs together. Bend the head backward, arching the back, and grasp the heels with the hands. Make a ninety-degree angle between the thighs and the calves. Inhale while going back, breathe slowly in position, then exhale while returning to the upright position.

TIME PERIOD: Can be done until the end of the seventh month.

BENEFITS: This asana tones the entire system, and helps strengthen apana vayu, the life-force energy responsible for delivery and all downward movement in the body.

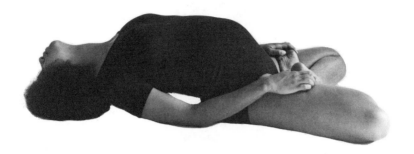

13. Fish

METHOD: Sit in the easy pose (simply crossing the legs in the ordinary way) or in the lotus pose. Take hold of the toes with the hands and lean backwards, arching the back so that the top of the head rests on the floor. Raise the chest as high as possible. Place your hands together in the prayer position on top of your chest. Breathe in as you enter the position—breathe deeply for several seconds, then exhale as you ease out of the pose.

ALTERNATE METHOD: Sit with the legs straight ahead. Now, instead of doing the asana in the Lotus or easy pose, simply arch the back in the same way, placing the hands underneath the buttocks for support.

TIME PERIOD: Can be done through the entire pregnancy.

BENEFITS: Relieves tension in the back and the chest, stretches and strengthens the back, and sends ample blood to the brain.

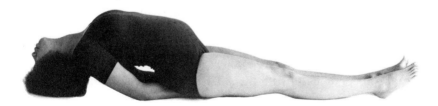

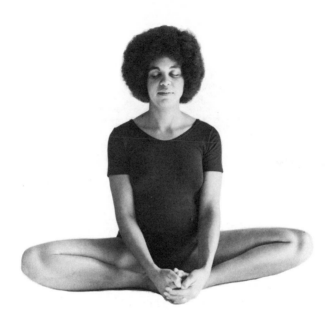

14. Shakti

METHOD: Sit on the floor. Bring the soles of the feet together, pushing the knees down to the floor. The heels should be as close as possible to the vagina. Place the hands on the knees, keeping the spine, neck, and head in a straight line. Concentrate in the "third eye"—the region between and behind the eyebrows. Breathe naturally. This position may be maintained for several minutes. It can also be done bobbing the legs up and down to achieve more flexibility.

TIME PERIOD: Can be done throughout the entire pregnancy.

BENEFITS: This asana, when done correctly, will elasticize the female sexual organs, thereby opening the birth canal and allowing for an easier delivery. Shakti is the Divine Mother, that aspect of God manifested by the feminine principle. The Shakti pose is of particular importance during pregnancy and can be done in conjunction with the Anal Sphincter Contraction (see pages 49–50).

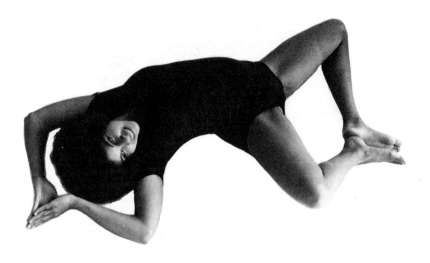

15. Tadpole

METHOD: Lie flat on the back. Place your hands together in the prayer position above your head. Bend the legs at the knees and bring the soles of the feet together. Then twist the lower body, including the legs, sideways, along with the upper body. Now twist to the other side. Move in this manner from left to right. Breathe gently as you move from side to side.

TIME PERIOD: Can be done through the entire pregnancy but should be stopped if there is discomfort.

BENEFITS: Strengthens all side muscles and stretches the spine, making it more elastic. Tones the nervous system and gives a general feeling of well-being.

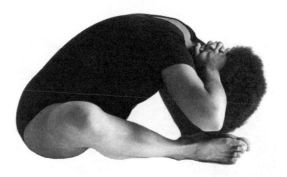

16. Star

METHOD: Sit as in the Shakti pose, but with the feet further away from the body (about one foot). Clasp the hands and place them on the forehead, then slowly bend forward, raising the knees slightly and transferring the clasped hands to the back of the head; try to touch the head to the feet. Breathe gently and deeply.

TIME PERIOD: Can be done throughout the entire pregnancy.

BENEFITS: Tones the abdominal area. Similar in effect to the Cat pose. Stretches the inside of the legs and helps to open the birth canal, making delivery easier.

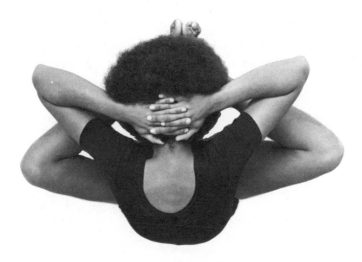

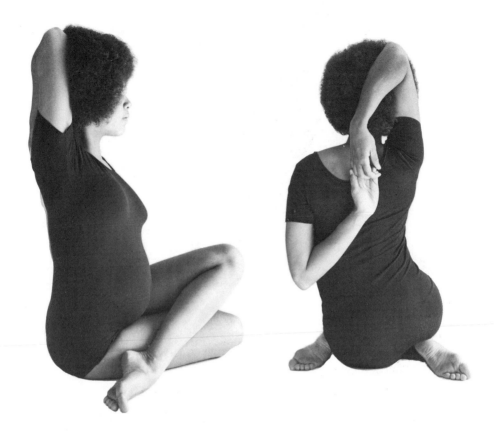

17. Cowhead

METHOD: Sit on the right leg, which is folded under; cross the left leg over the right and fold it similarly. Raise the right arm over the right shoulder, elbow bent so that the hand hangs down the back. Put the left hand behind the back and grasp the fingers of the right hand. Stretch, keeping the spine, neck, and head straight. Breathe deeply and slowly.

TIME PERIOD: Can be done through the entire pregnancy.

BENEFITS: Stretches the legs, arms, spine, and neck and helps to channel sexual energy.

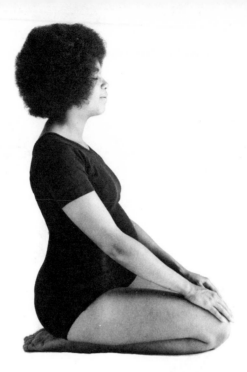

18. Nobleman

METHOD: Kneel and sit on the calves, with knees together. Place the hands on the knees. Keep arms and back straight, eyes focused on the tip of the nose. Breathe gently, deeply, and slowly. Hold this pose for 5 minutes.

TIME PERIOD: Can be done throughout the entire pregnancy.

BENEFITS: This asana is of immense benefit to the digestive system and is the only asana that can be done directly after eating. In pregnancy it will have a purifying effect and will help position the fetus correctly.

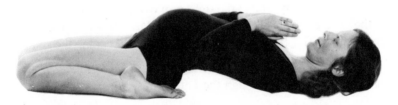

19. Lying Nobleman

METHOD: Sit as above. Inhale slowly and lie back on the calves. The knees should be together and touching the floor. Fold the hands on the chest in the prayer position. Breathe deeply and slowly in this position for about 30 seconds. Repeat twice.

TIME PERIOD: Can be done throughout the entire pregnancy.

BENEFITS: Stretches the legs, back, and abdominal area.

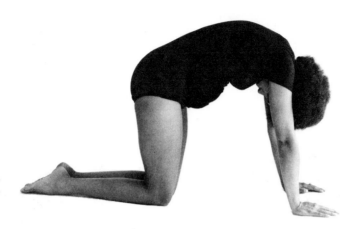

20. Cat

METHOD: Kneel on the floor on all fours. The hands should come straight down from the shoulders with the back straight. Inhale slowly through the mouth, making a hissing noise. At the same time, arch the back up like an angry cat and bend the head down until the chin presses the hollow of the neck. Gently stop the breath after inhalation for one or two seconds, while the chin presses the neck. Exhale slowly through the mouth while raising the head up as high as it will go and arching the back down in the opposite direction from the inhale position. Repeat two or three times.

TIME PERIOD: Can be done for the entire pregnancy.

BENEFITS: This asana is of particular benefit during pregnancy for it tones the entire system and facilitates delivery.

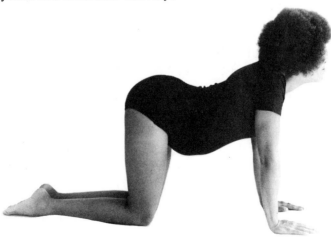

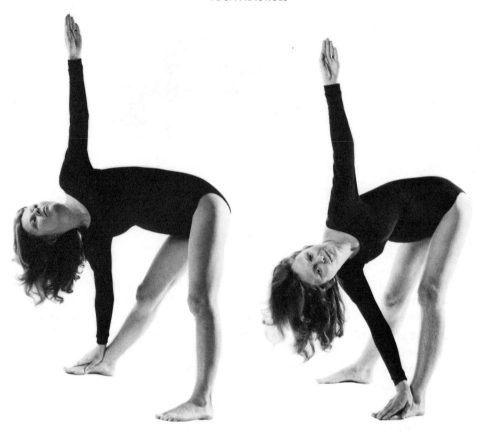

21. Standing Triangle, I and II

METHOD I: For Method I, stand with the feet a shoulder-width apart. Bending sideways, raise the right arm straight up and simultaneously touch the left hand to the left foot. Hold this position for 10 to 15 seconds, then straighten up. Then touch the right hand to the right foot, raising the left arm. Hold this position for 10 to 15 seconds.

METHOD II: Stand with the feet a shoulder-width apart. Bending the trunk and raising the left arm straight up, touch the right hand to the left foot. Hold this position for 10 to 15 seconds, breathing naturally. Now resume the standing posture. Repeat touching the left hand to the right foot. When in the posture, make sure that your arms make a 180-degree angle as shown.

TIME PERIOD: Can be done throughout the entire pregnancy.

BENEFITS: Stretches the legs, arms, and sides; increases the flow of blood to the brain; increases vitality and balance.

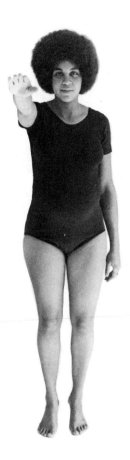

22. Palm Tree

METHOD: Stand erect, with toes together. Raise the right arm over the head with a swinging motion, while simultaneously standing on tiptoes. Pause, then come down and do the same with the left arm. Then raise both arms and stand on tiptoe. Inhale while raising the arms, hold the breath for two or three seconds while on tiptoes, then exhale as you bring the arms down. Do once with each arm and once with both arms.

TIME PERIOD: Can be done throughout the entire pregnancy.

BENEFITS: Like all exercises for balance, this asana develops the mind and makes it calm and one-pointed. Helps coordination and develops grace.

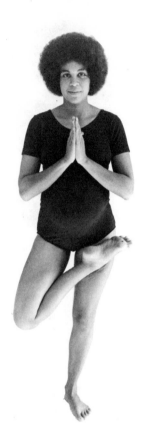

23. Tree

METHOD: Stand in balance, concentrating on a point on the wall in front of you. Raise the right leg, bending it at the knee and drawing it up over the left thigh. Raise both arms above the head, with palms together. Balance, keeping attention on the spot on the wall. Breathe naturally.

TIME PERIOD: Can be done during the entire pregnancy.

BENEFITS: Same as for Palm Tree pose.

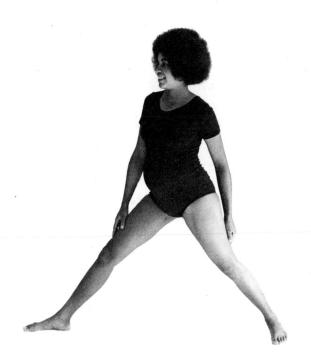

24. Standing Splits

METHOD: Stand with the legs as far apart as possible, then very gently proceed to "sit" between the outstretched legs. In the most advanced stage the legs would be completely flat on the floor.

TIME PERIOD: Can be practiced throughout the entire pregnancy.

BENEFITS: Stretches the birth canal and helps to eliminate impurities from the body.

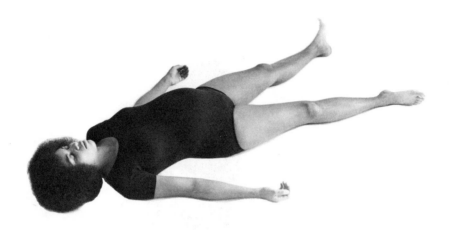

25. Corpse

METHOD: Lie flat on your back with your legs about one shoulder-width apart. Arms are about one foot from the body on each side, with palms up. Turn the head very slightly to the left or the right. *Relax completely.* Allow the breath to slow down until the entire system feels calm and serene. The Corpse pose is excellent after doing your daily yoga practice or after other asanas or breathing exercises, or at any time you feel tired. Focus the mind in a relaxed manner on the movement of breath, and be aware of any tenseness in the body; consciously relax these tensions. This asana is deceptively easy, for true relaxation is a very deep spiritual practice.

TIME PERIOD: Can be done throughout the entire pregnancy and should be practiced directly after each daily asana routine.

BENEFITS: Completely relaxes and energizes the system. The mind becomes free and calm. Practicing this asana can take the place of sleep if one can learn to completely relax without falling asleep. According to yoga texts, the Corpse pose practiced *properly* for a half-hour is equivalent, in terms of rest to the system, to six hours of sleep.

Suggested Program for Daily Practice

Up to the End of the Fourth Month

1. BREATHING

Alternate Nostril Breathing—10 rounds
Skull Shining—3 rounds of 20 breaths
Fire Cleansing—3 rounds of 20 pulls
Anal Sphincter Contractions—10 rounds

2. MEDITATION—one 15-minute session

3. ASANAS

Sun Salutation—3 times
Corpse
Shoulder Stand
Fish

Corpse

Half-Locust
Bow
Cobra
Nobleman
Lying Nobleman

Corpse

Camel
Half-Spinal Twist
Cowhead
Stretched Bow

Corpse

Standing Triangle
Palm Tree
Tree
Standing Splits

Corpse—5 minutes

From the Fifth Month to the End of the Seventh Month

1. BREATHING
Alternate Nostril Breathing
Skull Shining
Anal Sphincter Contraction (done in Shakti pose)
Piercing the Sun or The Cooling Breath,
    depending on hot or cold season

2. MEDITATION—one 20-minute session

3. ASANAS
Fish Pose

Camel
Wind-Releasing
Corpse
Shakti

Half-Spinal Twist
Cat
Cowhead

Corpse

Nobleman
Lying Nobleman

Standing Triangle
Standing Splits
Corpse

The Eighth and Ninth Months

1. BREATHING
Alternate Nostril Breathing
Skull Shining
Anal Sphincter Contraction (done in Shakti pose)
Piercing the Sun or The Cooling Breath,
    depending on hot or cold season.

2. MEDITATION—two 15-minute sessions a day

3. ASANAS

Do as many of the following asanas as you can. Pay particular attention to Shakti, Tadpole, Star, Cat, and Standing Splits. Do the asanas slowly but thoroughly. Rest in the Corpse pose in between each asana and at the end of each series.

Fish
Shakti
Tadpole
Star

Corpse

Cowhead
Nobleman
Lying Nobleman
Cat

Corpse

Standing Triangle
Palm Tree
Tree
Standing Splits

Corpse

7

DIET

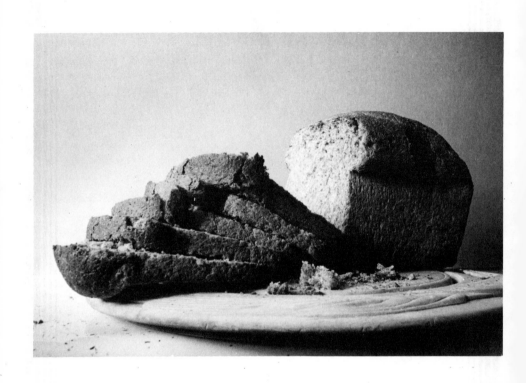

Diet is a preoccupation in our abundant society. Countless books are written and sold advocating everything from eating all raw fruit to consuming superhigh-protein diets. Each one is validated by impressive research and extensive study. It's enough to confuse a Ph.D. in nutrition!

Women often run to such books for advice when they find they are pregnant. The expectant mother is aware that her baby's nutrition is dependent on her eating habits. But her sincere desire to nourish the baby well can easily turn into a neurotic overemphasis on food. Relatives and friends can sometimes contribute to the confusion. Each has a pet theory which conflicts with a book or with someone else's theory or, most important, with your digestion. We hope our research will clarify and simplify your task of providing healthful food for yourself and your baby. Where there is weakness or disease, consult your physician for dietary advice or for medical treatment if necessary. This is especially true when using a program of vitamin supplements, since they should be taken in proportion to the special needs of pregnancy.

A Yoga Diet for Pregnancy

A yoga diet is based on a few essential rules:

1 The ideal yoga diet is vegetarian in obedience to the principle of noninjury. Eat a variety of vegetarian foods—grains, vegetables, fruits, nuts, legumes, and dairy products—to provide variety and balance.
2 Eat according to your digestion. If you cannot digest a food, it will not nourish your body. If a food, or a combination of foods, causes gas, indigestion, heartburn, or tiredness, refrain from eating it.
3 Eat calming food. Most vegetarian food is calming. Hot spices, garlic, onions, mushrooms, and flesh foods tend to stimulate the system. Use these sparingly.
4 Eat according to your nature. If you are prone to be overweight, avoid starchy, weight-producing food. If you tend to be underweight, you can eat larger quantities of starch.
5 Eat in harmony with the climate. Eat heavier, starchier foods in a cold climate. Eat lighter food in a warm climate.
6 Eat regular meals with several hours between eating. This enables food to be digested completely.

Yoga's recommendation of a vegetarian diet has been affirmed from another viewpoint. Studies in Canada and the United States show that women who are pregnant and wish to nurse should maintain a vegetarian diet. In 1975 the Environmental Protection Agency in Washington conducted a study of nursing mothers. The findings showed that the milk of 99 percent of these women contained concentrations of DDT and other pesticides which were unsafe for infant consumption. In 1977 the same agency conducted another study of vegetarian mothers. The results showed that these women had one-third to one-half the amount of DDT in their breast milk as meat-eating mothers.

CBC radio in Canada cited similar findings. They suggested over their national radio network that pregnant women who wished to nurse eat no more than one portion of fish per week, eat no meat, eat grains (which are generally grown without being treated with sprays), and wash their fruits and vegetables well. All toxic substances are to be avoided during pregnancy and nursing, for toxidity negatively affects the body, mind, and emotions, with the result that the baby suffers. In this connection, let us point out that cigarette smoke is also highly toxic. Although cigarettes are not a food, in a sense anything taken into the body is a kind of food. Numerous studies have shown that smoking has a debilitating effect on the growth of the developing child in the womb. Yoga considers smoking to be bad for the skin as well as the lungs and recommends that pregnant women breathe as much fresh, clean air as possible.

Protein

The concern for protein intake in America is so great that many people contemplating a vegetarian diet become anxious about the possibility of protein deficiency. Pregnant women are especially susceptible to these fears because their need for protein is so drastically increased during pregnancy. According to the Food and Nutrition Board of The National Research Council, National Academy of Sciences, in Washington, D.C., a woman's daily need for protein increases from 46 grams to 76 grams during pregnancy.

Fulfilling this need for protein does not need to be a complex matter. Be certain you take in about 60 grams of protein a day through high-protein sources. The other 16 grams you will get through incidental foods. There are small amounts of protein in almost everything you eat.

Here are some very simple ways of obtaining enough protein in one day.

Dairy Products

1) 2 cups cottage cheese   88 grams approximately

2) 1 cup cottage cheese   44
     1 quart buttermilk, yogurt, or milk   28
                                          72

3) 4 slices Swiss cheese   32
     1 quart milk   28
                                          60

Soy Products

1) 1 cup dry soybeans or soy grits   68 grams

2) ½ cup dry soybeans   34
     2 blocks of tofu (soybean curd)   16
     2 cups soy milk or yogurt   14
                                          64

3) 1 cup texturized vegetable protein   26 grams
     ½ cup soybeans   34
     1 cup soy milk or yogurt   8
                                          68

Whole Grains, Legumes, and Dairy Products

1) 1 peanut butter sandwich:
     2 tbsp. peanut butter   8 grams
     2 slices whole wheat bread   8
     1 serving lentils (⅓ cup dry)   13
     1 quart milk   28
                                          57

2) 1 cup gluten flour   85 grams

Gluten: A High Protein Food

A very concentrated form of protein is gluten, the substance which remains when the starch is removed from wheat flour. When prepared in the form of vegetarian "steaks," it has the chewy, salty texture and flavor of meat without any of the toxins or the taking of animal life.

Gluten Steaks: Recipe 1

GLUTEN

8 cups hard wheat or high-gluten wheat flour
2 cups water

GRAVY

1 quart water
½ cup tamari soy sauce
2 tsp. ground cumin
2 tsp. ground coriander
½ tsp. black pepper
2 tbsp. flour

1 Mix the water into the flour until a dough is formed.
2 Knead for 30 minutes. Kneading develops the gluten. When the dough is sufficiently kneaded, it will bounce back when punched.
3 Place the ball of dough into a large bowl of cold water, enough to completely cover the ball.
4 Let the dough soak for 2 hours.
5 Knead the dough under the water. This will separate the starch from the gluten. The water will become milky as the starch is eliminated. As you knead, be careful to keep the gluten intact.
6 Change the water when it becomes very milky. Change it several times until the water stays clear when you knead the ball. (If you don't get all the starch separated from the gluten, your "steaks" will taste like soggy bread instead of chewy "meat.")
7 The gluten should now be very elastic and stringy. Pull pieces off the whole and stretch them into ¼- to ½-inch-thick irregular shapes.
8 Place the steaks in a broth made from the water, tamari soy sauce, cumin, coriander, and pepper. Cook for one-half hour over medium heat.
9 Make a paste of 2 tbsp. flour and ¼ cup cold water. Add to the mixture and cook for 10 minutes.
10 Serve when a gravy has been formed. Excess portions can be frozen.

Gluten Steaks: Recipe 2

Many health food stores carry 80 percent gluten flour. Making gluten from this flour is a simple way to provide large quantities of protein.

1 Gradually stir water into the gluten flour until a stringy, stiff dough is formed.
2 Knead the dough into the form of a roll.
3 Slice this roll into ¼-inch rounds.
4 Place in broth as described in recipe 1 and boil lightly for 45 minutes.
5 Make a paste of 2 tbsp. flour and ¼ cup cold water. Add this to the broth and gluten.
6 Serve when a gravy has formed.

Vitamins and Minerals

The subject of the multitude of vitamins and minerals, their nutritional functions and sources, is far beyond the scope of this book. Therefore, our discussion of vitamins will be limited to those few vitamins and minerals which are required in substantially increased quantities during pregnancy.

The vitamins and minerals to be considered are folic acid, calcium, phosphorus, magnesium, and iron. Your need for folic acid will double during pregnancy. The requirements for calcium and phosphorus increase by two-thirds. Phosphorus is increased by 50 percent. Iron is needed in varying amounts depending on the individual's tendency to be anemic. Other vitamins and minerals are also needed in larger quantities, but the increases are small relative to these five essential pregnancy nutrients.

Folic acid is abundantly available in vegetables. It is found in high concentrations in leafy green vegetables, fruit, brewer's (or nutritional) yeast, milk, cheese, and whole grains. Eating fruit with breakfast and large green salads at lunch and dinner should satisfy your need for folic acid. You will be getting additional quantities from the milk, cheese, and whole grains that you take in the course of your day. Brewer's yeast is a good supplement to take during pregnancy if you can digest it. If it causes indigestion and gas, even in small quantities, then don't use it.

Calcium can be obtained in large quantities from almonds, raw kelp, Swiss cheese, sesame seeds, turnip greens, and whole wheat bread. Of these, raw kelp and sesame seeds have by far the largest concentrations of calcium. Kelp can be obtained in powder form and sprinkled generously on salads,

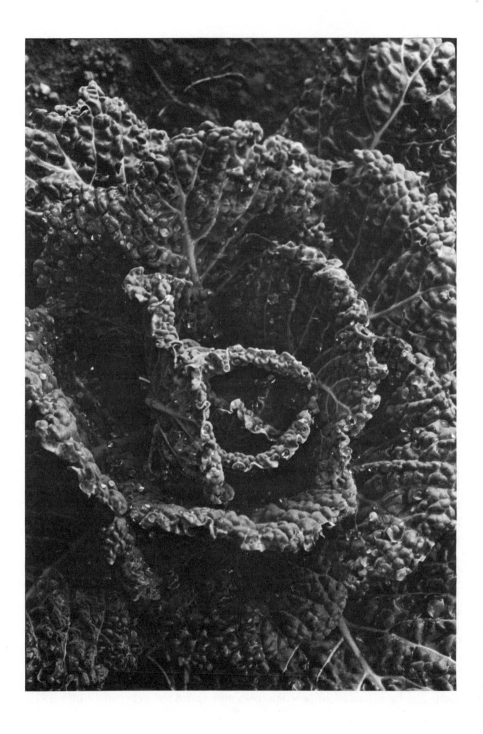

vegetables, and grains. Tahini, made from ground sesame seeds, provides a good base when mixed with lemon and water for creamy salad dressing. You can vary the seasoning and use it generously on your twice-daily salads. In addition, eating a few almonds with every meal will increase your calcium intake.

Phosphorus is best supplied by wheat germ and brewer's yeast. Wheat germ can be taken quite palatably and in substantial quantity in yogurt with fruit for breakfast. Again, whether you can use brewer's yeast depends on your digestive power. Other good sources of phosphorus are toasted whole wheat bread, Swiss cheese, cashews, oats, peanuts, lentils, and sesame and sunflower seeds.

Magnesium is found abundantly in wheat germ, crude wheat bran, soybeans, peanuts, blackstrap molasses, cashews, and almonds. Since many of these foods have also been mentioned as being high in other important nutrients needed during pregnancy, their use will inevitably provide the quantities of magnesium necessary for health.

Although the quantity of iron required for a healthy pregnancy may vary from woman to woman, the risk of iron-deficiency anemia is always a possibility to be avoided. Blackstrap molasses contains an extremely high concentration of iron (twice as much as found in beef liver by equal weight). Molasses and milk is a pleasant way to take protein, magnesium, and iron in combination. (Blackstrap molasses is also a laxative.) Brewer's yeast (if digestible) and sesame seeds are also excellent sources of iron.

If you can digest them, natural vitamin supplements can provide extra assurance, since some of the foods you eat may have lost some nutritional value through being shipped over long distances or stored for long periods. However, be sure to read the label before you buy a supplement if you wish to observe seriously the principle of noninjury: some products contain minerals derived from animal bones. You may also prefer tablets to capsules, which contain gelatin made from animal remains.

Sample Vegetarian Menus

To make the preceding nutritional information more practical, we provide a few sample daily menus. By following these suggestions and/or making your own conscious plans for daily eating, you will satisfy your need for good nutrition throughout pregnancy.

Day 1

BREAKFAST:

1 cup cottage cheese with wheat germ, fruit, almonds, and cashews.

LUNCH:

1 12-ounce glass of milk with blackstrap molasses
1 Swiss cheese sandwich on whole wheat bread (several pieces of cheese)
1 salad with sesame tahini dressing, sprinkled with kelp and alfalfa sprouts.

DINNER:

1 serving of texturized vegetable protein chunks in gravy
1 green salad with tahini dressing and kelp and alfalfa sprouts
1 cooked vegetable
1 serving of grains—brown rice, bulgar, millet, or kasha

BEDTIME:

1 cup warm milk with blackstrap molasses

Day 2

BREAKFAST:

oatmeal with wheat germ, sunflower seeds, cashews, almonds, and fruit,
  served with 1 cup milk

LUNCH:

1 cup yogurt seasoned with vegetable broth to use as a dip
cut-up carrots, green peppers, and lettuce for dipping
1 serving of lentil soup

DINNER:

1 serving of gluten steak
1 salad with tahini dressing, kelp, and alfalfa sprouts
1 cooked vegetable
1 serving of grains or potatoes

BEDTIME:

1 cup warm milk with blackstrap molasses

Day 3

BREAKFAST:

1 cup yogurt with wheat germ, cashews, almonds, and fruit

LUNCH:

1 large salad with grated yellow cheese, kelp, alfalfa sprouts, and vinegar-and-oil dressing
1 serving of corn chowder made with milk

DINNER:

1 serving of soybean casserole with sesame seeds*
1 cucumber salad with yogurt dressing
1 cooked vegetable
1 serving of grains

BEDTIME:

1 cup warm milk with blackstrap molasses

Day 4

BREAKFAST:

1 Swiss cheese sandwich on whole wheat toast
1 cup warm milk with blackstrap molasses
1 fruit
1 serving of roasted almonds and cashews

LUNCH:

1 bowl of tomato, navy bean, or vegetable soup
½ cup cottage cheese
1 green salad with tahini dressing, kelp, and alfalfa sprouts
whole wheat crackers

DINNER:

1 serving of lentil loaf
1 serving of grains
1 cooked vegetable
1 Greek salad with feta cheese

BEDTIME:

1 cup warm milk with blackstrap molasses

---

*See *Diet for a Small Planet* and *The Vegetarian Alternative* for recipes for this casserole and the lentil loaf listed below; see Suggested Reading List, p. 148.

Day 5

BREAKFAST:

granola (with sesame seeds, cashews, almonds, and toasted wheat germ)
  with fresh fruit, served in 1 cup milk, yogurt, or buttermilk

LUNCH:

1 peanut butter sandwich on whole wheat bread
1 cup buttermilk
1 portion tahini dip (tahini, water, lemon, and salt)
cut-up carrots for dipping

DINNER:

1 cup lentil soup
1 generous serving of tofu (soybean curd)
1 serving of grains
1 cooked vegetable
1 salad with alfalfa sprouts, kelp, sunflower seeds, and lemon-and-oil
  dressing

BEDTIME:

1 cup warm milk with molasses

8

YOGA
PRACTICE
AFTER THE
BIRTH

Resuming Breathing Exercises

The first two weeks after a child's birth should be a time of restful enjoyment of the new relationship between mother and child. It is best not to follow any structured exercise during this period.

After two weeks one exercise becomes extremely helpful to the healing and strengthening of the female organs: the Anal Sphincter Contraction (see page 49). It can be practiced in any sitting position several times a day providing you have not eaten within the previous two hours. To get the most out of this exercise, practice five to ten rounds of contractions three times a day. No additional breathing exercises need be practiced until six weeks after the birth.

When your baby is six weeks old, a full routine of breathing exercises (as described in chapter 4) may be resumed. These will, again, become a powerful tool for centering the mind as a prelude to meditation.

Maintaining Meditation

During the first weeks and early months after a child is born, it is not always possible to maintain the same meditation schedule that was practiced before the birth. The baby's needs for food, comfort, and diaper changes are the priorities in your life now. Meditation practice should be continued, however, if at all possible. Practicing meditation will enable you to maintain a restful state of mind so that you can attend to the common problems of babyhood—colic, diaper rash, teething, wakefulness—without being upset. In addition, meditation will help you to sleep and rest so that you can recover from the exhaustion which hard labor can cause.

You can make a firm resolution to stop everything and meditate as soon as your baby falls asleep in the morning. This sometimes takes an extra measure of discipline. You may have to leave the half-done dishes or housework until later. You may find it necessary to sit in meditation with your baby in your arms. The important thing is to maintain a commitment to the practice of daily sitting and stilling the mind.

Resuming Asanas after Six Weeks

The first six weeks after birth should be devoted to rest, sleep, and gentle relaxing activity. No strain or exercise should be exerted by the body. As a result of your prenatal exercises, your body will regain its shape and strength within a few weeks. Rest, rather than exercise, is what you need to recover from childbirth.

After six weeks, the internal organs have returned to normal. At this time you are ready to begin a daily routine of asanas again. It is not necessary to follow a particular routine of postnatal exercises. You can include any asanas which you enjoy or feel a need to practice. The general rules for creating a balanced and beneficial program are the same as the rules for creating such a program before pregnancy. You may again add inverted poses to your program. We have included a program which may be helpful. Remember that the peace of mind and health of the body created by yoga practice is as beneficial in your life now as it was during pregnancy.

1. BREATHING

Alternate Nostril Breathing—10 rounds
Skull Shining—3 rounds of 20 breaths
Fire Cleansing—3 rounds of 20 pulls
Anal Sphincter Contractions—10 rounds

2. MEDITATION—one 15-minute session

3. ASANAS

Sun Salutation—3 times

Corpse

Shoulder Stand
Fish

Corpse

Half-Locust
Bow
Cobra
Nobleman
Lying Nobleman

Corpse

Camel
Half-Spinal Twist
Cowhead
Stretched Bow

Corpse

Standing Triangle
Palm Tree
Tree
Standing Splits

Corpse—5 minutes

DEVELOPMENT OF THE EMBRYO AND BIRTH

9

THE EMBRYO'S GROWTH INTO A HUMAN BEING

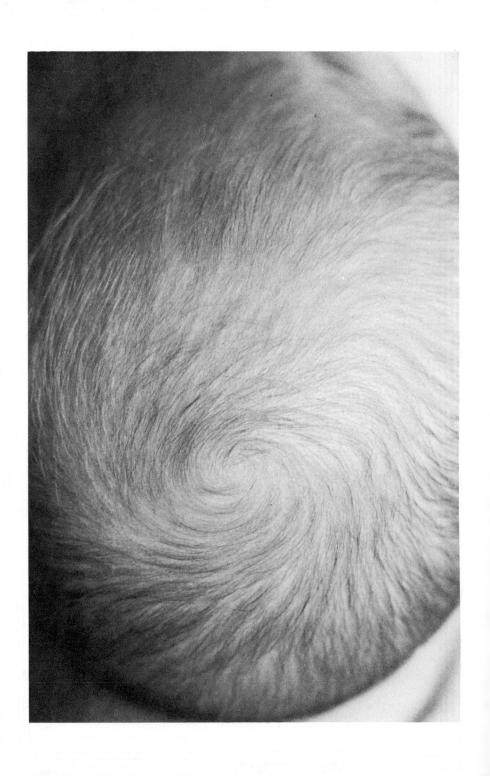

This explanation of the child's development in the womb is not a recounting of the fetus's physical growth. It is a description of the stages at which the human attributes of soul, spiritual heart, mind, and intellect enter the being. As these nonphysical qualities become active, the experience and nature of the child change. We share this information so that mothers and fathers can gain a greater understanding of what is happening within the woman's body. By understanding how and when these human qualities develop, you can respond to your baby's changing needs.

We are grateful to our teacher, Baba Hari Dass, for giving us this information. He said, "Some old saints in India told me." However, we did find that what he taught us about the mental, emotional, and spiritual development of the fetus is affirmed by several classic Ayurvedic medical texts.* Ayurveda, the ancient medical system of India, is considered a sister science to the science of yoga and is recognized as the mother of all of the classical Oriental medical systems, including the Chinese, Japanese, and Tibetan.

A New Life Begins: Conception

A new life begins with the act of lovemaking. When the primal desire to reproduce is strong, and when the physical and subtle ingredients necessary to the process are harmonized, a being is conceived.

The conception of a person, according to yoga, is the bringing of a soul from the subtle, or nonphysical, realm into physical existence. According to the theory of reincarnation, a soul is brought back to the world by a process of vibrational attraction to the parents. This is a natural, spontaneous occurrence caused by the cumulative effect of the desires and habits of the mother, father, and child, established in previous relationships in former lives. These desires, habits, and tendencies of the parents, called samskaras, act much like a magnet drawing the soul into the mother's womb.

The First Month: The Soul

According to yoga theory, the human body is composed of five elements called earth, water, fire, air, and ether. (Ether may be defined as the space within which the other elements operate.) At conception the elements con-

*For those interested in further study, both the Sushruta Samhita and the Charaka Samhita go into some detail on the subject.

tained in the sexual fluids of the father and the mother combine to form a gelatinous substance. In the first period of approximately four weeks, a jellylike mass which has no recognizable human characteristics is formed. During this time, heating and cooling activities and impulses inside the mother's body gradually begin to mold the five elements, which have now combined into a human form. On the twenty-second day of this shaping, forming, condensing process, the soul enters the still jellylike body.

The Second Month through the Third Month: Formation of the Body

In the second month the five elements interact with each other and the body of the child becomes solid. The five elements begin to take on the characteristics of a human body.

Earth is represented in the human body by solid, immobile substances such as bone, which provides support for the body.

Water is represented by all the fluids and soft matter in the body: lymph, blood, alkaline mucous secretions, semen, sexual secretions, and fat. These components bind the body together.

Fire is represented by heat in the body as generated by acid digestive fluids and other heat-producing secretions.

Air is represented by the nervous activity of the body. This nervous activity is responsible for movement and sensation.

Ether is represented by the various networks which pervade the entire body, including the nervous system and the veins and arteries.

Throughout the gestation period, these five elements grow, mature, and interact so that the fetus becomes increasingly recognizable as a human body.

The Fourth Month: The Spiritual Heart

Four months after conception the baby is a physically well-formed human being, though only eight inches long. At this time, says yoga, the spiritual heart of the small infant becomes active. The spiritual heart is the seat of consciousness, the source of feeling and emotion; it is not the physical heart which pumps the blood. The mother now possesses two seats of consciousness within her being, her own and her baby's.

From this time until after the infant is born, the baby's desires are felt by the mother as though they were her own. The infant wants certain smells, tastes, and feelings which are a reflection of his needs as he grows.* At this stage, the mother has a responsibility to satisfy the urges that she may feel, no matter how unusual they may be—for a baked potato in the middle of the night or rock 'n' roll music first thing in the morning. So long as the mother carries the baby's seat of consciousness within her, she must set aside her own prejudices and be responsive.

Here we are making a distinction between instinctive *needs* for substances that aid the physical growth of the child (such as certain nutrients in food) and *desires* for certain impressions that the soul needs to experience for the fulfillment of its karma (given that the soul of the child is not a "new" soul but has already accumulated a burden of samskaras from previous lifetimes). This explains why the mother should indulge the whims, as it were, of the child even if the child desires something that the mother, with her fully developed sense of discrimination, would not ordinarily choose—such as meat. The child has not the capacity to fulfill its own needs at this point and depends utterly on the mother. It cannot know, for example, that eating meat violates the rule of noninjury; it can only sense the fulfillment or frustration of its needs. Thus, the fulfillment of its desires by the mother is an act of compassion and love that helps the baby to learn trust and faith that needs will be met.

The Fifth Month: The Mind

At five months the baby awakens from his subconscious state and begins to develop manas (the individual mind which has the power and faculty of attention). The infant is now affected by the thoughts of the mother. Therefore, if the mother turns her mind toward positivity and concentrates on cultivating spirituality, her child's mental processes can be set in motion in a wonderful way. Because mother and baby share the same environment so intensely, when the mother feeds her mind with beautiful thoughts through devotional stories, spiritual teachings, or humorous writings, her baby will be affected likewise.

---

*We are following the convention of using the masculine pronouns *he* and *his* to refer to the child whose sex is unknown, in order to avoid the awkwardness of "he or she" and "his or her."

The Sixth Month

In the sixth month the infant's intellect (buddhi) begins to awaken. Now the baby is fully human, able to experience and differentiate between the pleasure of comfort and the pain of discomfort. These experiences are felt as if in a dream state rather than in the way experiences affected the baby before the intellect developed.

The Seventh and the Eighth Months: Maturation

The last three months before birth are a maturing period. During this time the child experiences physical discomfort. He is "squished" into a small space which seems to grow smaller daily. No longer can he move around, floating freely in space. This confinement is both painful and pleasurable. Mother moves suddenly or awkwardly and the baby's whole body is contorted. Yet there is support and warmth and rhythm. The baby has no choice but to accept the situation. In this way nature is nurturing the quality of contentment in the child. The baby is in no way being harmed. The unchangeable realities of life cannot hurt; they can only strengthen. The words of Baba Hari Dass may be helpful in understanding the child's experience in the womb when conditions have become physically confining: "It is useless to regret that the child feels pain or pleasure inside the womb, because it's a law of nature that everyone has to pass through these stages. God has made a perfect system of nature so that everything is controlled. If suffering comes, then the strength to tolerate it also comes. If a child in the womb suffers pain, then definitely some kind of pranic energy will develop which will give strength to tolerate it."

During this time the baby is a physically, emotionally, and spiritually formed human being. The experiences of the child now have tremendous effect on his development. Your own physical, emotional, and mental state constitutes the environment your child is growing in. However, your baby is not merely a sponge which absorbs your state of being without consciousness. The six-month-old baby in the womb is a being with his own desires, thoughts, and emotions. You too are affected by your child's being and nature. In a sense, during the last three months before birth your relationship is that between two equal human beings contained in one body. It is no wonder that spiritual teachers have often called the relationship between mother and child the highest human relationship.

124

The Ninth Month: Approaching Birth

As we have said, from six months on, the child has been finding himself increasingly confined in the small space of the womb. In the ninth month sensations similar to earth tremors are added to the child's experience. Imagine this: It's night. You're in a very tiny room, asleep in a snug sleeping bag. Suddenly, the whole building trembles. It feels as though the hand of God had picked up the building, given it a good shake, and then set the building down again. The infant has this kind of experience throughout the last month of his stay in the womb. He is conscious now and reacts to experience with emotion. Depending on his nature, this event may terrorize, excite, please, or dismay the small person. Whatever the child's reaction, he will become accustomed to this sensation. Again, the child will learn patience, endurance, and strength. He is coming closer to an even greater lesson in endurance—the pain-pleasure of labor and birth.

10

GIVING
BIRTH

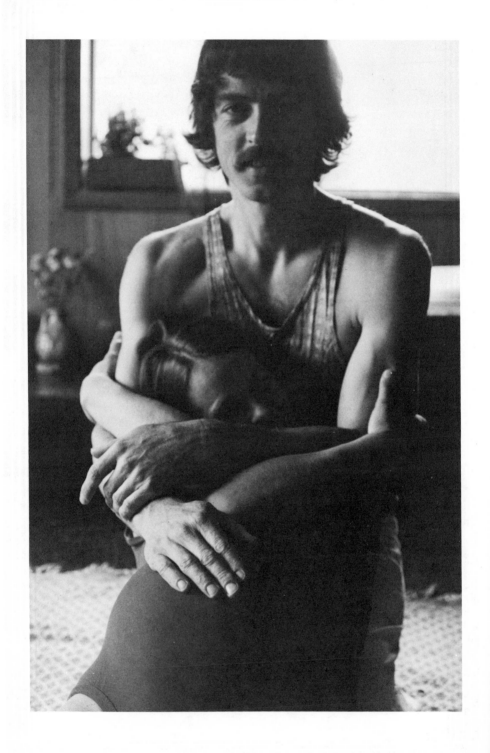

The Three Stages of Labor

Labor is unique for every woman. You won't know how it is for you until it's over. Then it will be a vivid memory which gives you a greater knowledge of your strength as a human being.

However, in preparing psychologically for labor, there are likely patterns to consider. By understanding these patterns in advance, you and your husband can appreciate the emotional rhythm of giving birth. Being prepared can make the birth a transcendent experience.

Your labor will likely proceed in three emotional and physical stages. At stage one, contractions are mild and come every fifteen to thirty minutes. You will probably enjoy human contact, talking, and quiet activity. Stage two is the height of labor when contractions occur five to two minutes apart. You need extreme concentration and stillness in order to maintain calm control during this stage. Stage three is the final pushing stage. You will probably be alert, aware, and more outgoing.

The Subtle Forces That Aid Childbirth

There are two subtle energy forces, or pranas, which aid during childbirth. In yoga these forces are called anant vayu and apana vayu. As mentioned in chapter 1, anant vayu functions throughout pregnancy. It contributes to morning sickness in the first three months and brings about heightened sense awareness, exhilaration, and inspiration throughout the remainder of pregnancy. During labor anant vayu functions to intoxicate the mother and thus counteracts the pain of childbirth. When labor begins, a surge of energy flows toward the heart and head, awakening love and inspiration. This flow of energy becomes stronger as labor progresses. Thus, a woman who calmly lets nature's forces aid her in pregnancy feels greater and greater confidence and is able to withstand the increase in pain. This effect of anant vayu should not be confused with a feeling of being "spaced out" or in a stupor. It is rather an increased awareness of the needs of the situation and how to respond to those needs most appropriately.

The second force at work during labor is apana vayu. This prana aids all downward-flowing functions in the body, including urination and defecation. During labor, apana vayu has the function of pushing the baby down the birth canal. Accordingly, yoga for pregnancy emphasizes practices which strengthen this energy.

During labor a strong and healthy flow of apana vayu makes for the steady downward movement of the child. The breathing pattern during labor influences the flow of apana vayu and thus the progress of labor. Therefore, yoga teaches breathing techniques which develop apana vayu during the gestation period, in preparation for the actual birth, and for labor, which causes apana vayu to flow downward.

The help of anant vayu and apana vayu can be strengthened or minimized during labor, depending on the expectant mother's state of mind. Serenity is the quality needed to enable these forces to work effectively. An agitated or frightened woman will not be able to feel the intoxicating effects of anant vayu and will thereby inhibit the smooth downward flow of apana vayu.

Calmness and Control through Breathing

According to yoga, breath has the ability to regulate the state of mind. Calm, deep breathing produces the serenity necessary for a controlled natural childbirth. A simple but effective method of yoga breathing is especially recommended for use during contractions. To maintain this breathing pattern throughout both light and heavy contractions takes will power and self-discipline. The impulse to lose control must be silenced.

When a contraction begins, sit or lie in any comfortable position. Breathe in gently, slowly, and deeply through the nose. The breath will cause the abdomen to push out slightly. Then exhale slowly and gently through the mouth. The lips can be extended slightly; this causes the air to be expelled more slowly. As the air is released, the stomach is contracted slightly. This is a gentle breathing method. It should not feel forced or unnatural.

This breathing pattern stimulates both anant vayu and apana vayu. The slow, gentle nature of the breathing soothes the mind and stabilizes the emotions, and this in turn allows anant vayu to have a strong and positive effect. The downward flow of apana vayu is also strengthened by this slow, deep breathing. The deepness of the breath into the abdomen promotes the action of this energy, thus causing the downward flow which helps the child progress through the birth canal. The slowness of the breath establishes a pattern in which the exhalation is lengthened. Ideally the exhalation should be twice as long as the inhalation. This rhythm need not be forced. It will establish itself naturally in due course if the breath is calm. The length of the exhalation is important because it is directly related to the strength of apana vayu's downward flow. The longer and steadier the outgoing breath, the stronger and steadier the downward movement of the baby will be.

This breathing pattern is also beneficial for the long hours of labor because it energizes and revitalizes the body and mind. Slow, deep breathing will not tire the pregnant woman as will more erratic types of breathing.

Relaxing during Light Labor

During the initial period of light labor, it is probable that you'll feel nervous about labor. Even if you have given birth previously, your present labor is a new and unknown territory.

As contractions begin, you will find them a strange sensation. The first contractions may well be like intense shivers of slight electric impulses. They seem to reach out and touch the whole body from head to fingertips and toes. When these contractions come, feel them completely. Use deep, slow breathing as a means of accepting them. After a few hours you will be familiar with the rhythm of your labor. As strangeness vanishes, so will fear.

When fear is gone, the quality of the pain changes. The force with which the contractions take over your body increases gradually, but they are no longer accompanied by panic. At this point a contraction can be likened to a powerful wave that sweeps you into another dimension. In that dimension there is only pressure and breath; all else vanishes. For me this wave of pain was more than an analogy. Between contractions I felt I was resting on a beach. Each time a contraction started I had a vision of being grabbed by a wave and being transported by its rolling motion to a place where I was completely unaware of the people or the sounds around me. I was conscious only of the movement within my body. Breathing slowly, my body rocked to an internal rhythm. When one contraction passed, I explained to my husband, "I'm just learning to ride the waves."

It's an amazing thing about labor contractions: the sensations come in an instant and disappear just as quickly. There is total relief between each. From the very beginning of labor, use the moments of relief between contractions to rejuvenate yourself. Rejuvenation occurs through relaxation. If you melt into a feeling of appreciation for the moment of stillness in between, then the contractions will not frighten or tire you. If you are constantly anticipating the contractions, fear will be the dominent mood. This fear can keep you from having the rest needed for prolonged labor.

Thoughts and feelings like "It's about time," "I'm going to see my baby

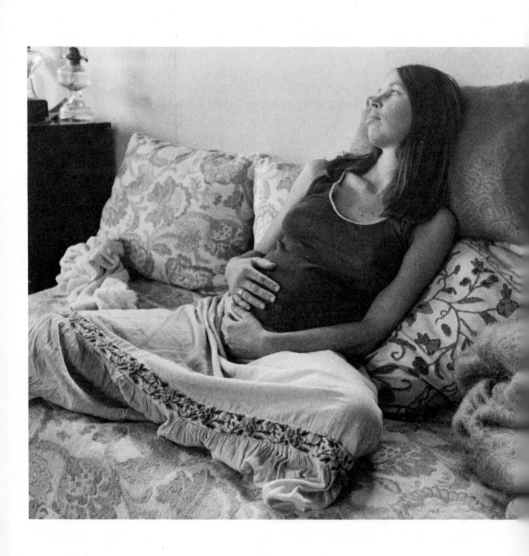

today," "Will I be strong enough?," "God, this is weird," "I'm scared," and so on may keep you from relaxing between contractions in the initial stage of labor. Sharing your feelings with your husband may be a way of eliminating nervous thought activity. Tell him how you feel and what you're thinking, or what you need. When a contraction comes, stop talking, feel the sensation, then go on communicating. Explain the feeling of the contraction to him. Listening to his feelings of concern, excitement, anxiety, will help you to forget your own preoccupations. The words between you at this stage are a wonderful vehicle for the special intimacy that is shared in giving birth.

If your feelings of excitement and anticipation are relieved early in labor, sleeping is probably the best thing to do between contractions. Sleep will conserve your strength. Most of us, however, are wide awake at the beginning of labor, and enforced rest might only increase agitation. In that case, quiet, soothing activities may be more calming than forced stillness. Taking a bath, lying in the sun, watching the stars, and reading inspiring books are simple activities which help you to relax in between the initial light contractions.

Staying Calm during Heavy Labor

As contractions progress, you will need to concentrate more. You'll probably want stillness and a comfortable place to be. You may even want complete quiet and solitude. To concentrate on your breath, to control your emotions, to remain relaxed, to ride the waves of pain without resistance require intense concentration.

Your husband can provide reassurance at this intense time. Tell him what your need is. He can be with you in stillness, breathing with you and meditating between contractions. If you want him to hold your hand, to stroke your back, to reassure you, then let him know. But if you need isolation, then tell him.

The strength required by you at this stage is obvious. You will be totally involved. The word *labor* is appropriate. You will be working very hard. Every few moments your body will be gripped by an intense and totally consuming sensation. This stage of labor is a wonderful challenge. It is an opportunity to achieve inner strength through self-control and to understand the true meaning of surrender in the spiritual sense.

A vivid memory from my own labor may help to illustrate this point. When I was experiencing this intense stage of labor, my mind recalled an experience my husband and I had had a few months earlier. We had been at a zen sesshin—a kind of meditation retreat. Our practice consisted mainly of staring at a wall while breathing slowly for twelve hours a day, for eight days. After two days I was tired; my legs ached; I was, in a word, sick of the whole boring experience. Then I told myself, "Well, you're not going to get out of this, so you might as well accept it." With this realization, my whole experience of the meditation changed. Now I continued meditating with fresh energy, directing my mind away from the thoughts of protest and complaint. Simply accepting my condition had somehow made the condition itself change.

Lying on my bed after an hour of heavy labor, feeling slightly irritated about the whole boring business, I remembered the zen sesshin. My mind again said, "You're not going to get out of this, so you might as well accept it." Again my experience changed. I began to drift into half-sleep between contractions. I felt a floating sensation. A sense of calm encircled my being. During contractions, my consciousness was totally consumed by the sensations (which I cannot call pain). My slow breathing continued and I was transported to a space beyond time and beyond sense awareness. I was, quite miraculously, enjoying the experience I had been loathing a short time earlier.

Pushing during Labor

The final or pushing stage of labor is the most dynamic and, for most women, the least painful part of childbirth. During this stage you will likely be seized by an overwhelming desire to push. This desire brings with it a surge of energy enabling you to concentrate fully on the demands of this stage.

Your breathing will probably change greatly during the pushing contractions. When you push, you naturally retain an inhaled breath. When it becomes necessary to exhale and again inhale, you will do so quite quickly since you are unable to maintain the same pressure while breathing.

Very near the time of birth, your doctor or midwife may ask you to stop bearing down. The purpose of this request is to slow the birth of your child in order to prevent tearing of the vaginal opening. At this time, short "blow" breaths through the mouth will alleviate the impulse to bear down. Thirty-five to forty of these breaths can be taken in one minute. The purpose of this breath is to keep from bearing down, not to alleviate pain. It should be used only at this stage if required. During other stages of labor it will cause emotional agitation and thirst.

Your Child Is Born

The atmosphere becomes electric just before a child is born. The moments of birth are so profound that the mind is stilled by the vision of the unfolding events.

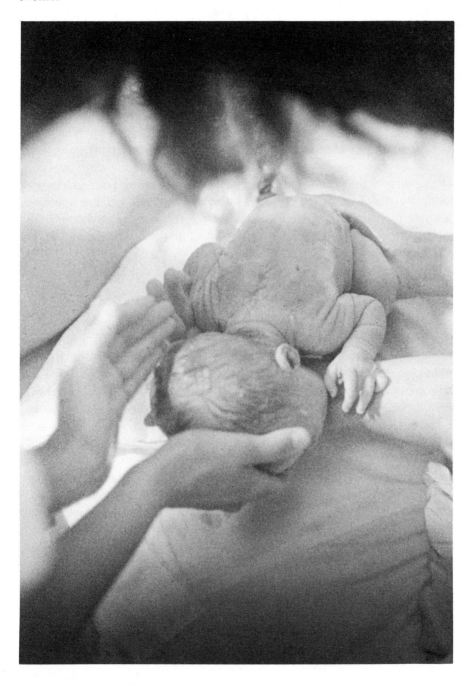

The emergence of the child's head causes onlookers to gasp involuntarily. The mother's pushing, as well as the stretching of her vagina, are so intense, so concentrated, and so prolonged that when in one push the entire head comes into the world it is literally breathtaking (particularly for the father). There is the child—half emerged, alive, making sounds and responding.

A moment later, the baby's body slithers out. The body is not forced through a barrier like the head was, and it simply slides out. The body is clean and shining. Suddenly an utterly perfect synthesis of husband and wife is before you. The moment is natural and comfortable, but very special, because there are no thoughts beyond the present. You are together here and now, responding appropriately to the moment. It is utterly simple.

Being a Mother: The Importance of Imprinting

After giving birth, you feel a natural and intense need to hold and look at your baby. You feel, as do all mothers who are conscious while giving birth, that this first time of closeness creates an indelible bond. You somehow know that this intimate beginning will stretch into the future and affect your whole relationship with your family.

Behavioral scientists, pediatricians, and doctors are now confirming with research what many mothers have known instinctively. Some of the most extensive research in the field of imprinting has been done by Dr. Marshall Klaus, a pediatrician at Case Western Reserve University School of Medicine. Imprinting is learning that occurs rapidly in the first moments after birth. The mother's behavior as well as the child's is influenced by imprinting. Dr. Klaus's research shows that a mother's responses to her child are established in the moments, hours, and days immediately following birth. Dr. Klaus found that mothers who were given their naked babies immediately after birth and were then left undisturbed for five to sixteen hours made similar, apparently instinctual affectionate gestures toward their children. They stroked, caressed, and communicated with them in predictable and similar ways. For two years following birth, the mothers who fulfilled this early instinctual contact were more patient and loving toward their children than mothers who were separated from their babies. The "imprinted" mothers explained things to their children and comforted them when they were upset. The rapport was greater.*

*Birth and Family Journal, vol. 1, no. 3 (Summer 1974).

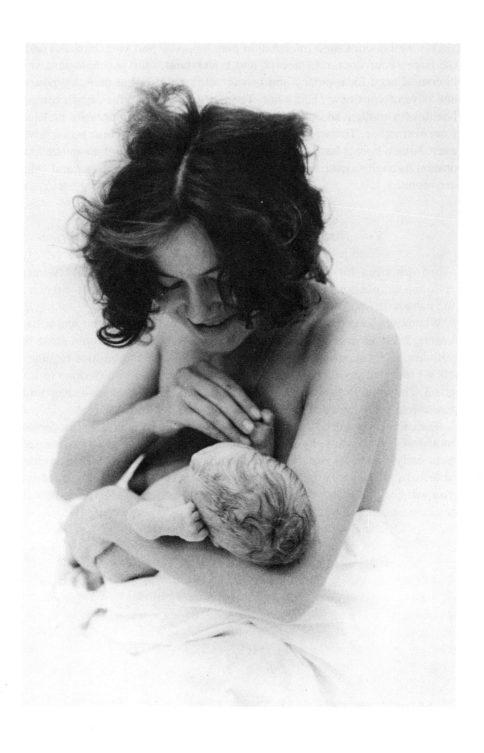

This well-documented information may help you and your husband and, we hope, your doctor to accept and understand your psychological and biological need for intimacy and privacy during those first minutes, hours, and days of your new child's life. There are, however, times when for the health of a mother and/or child, a newborn infant is temporarily isolated from his mother. This event is no doubt emotionally difficult for both. However, human beings have the ability to overcome this temporary initial separation through sharing love, warmth, and closeness when mother and child are reunited.

Nursing: A Restful Relationship

When this need for closeness is satisfied, it does not go away. A deep spiritual, natural bond is established and is further enhanced when you nurse the baby with your own milk.

When my daughter was nursing (which she did for over two and a half years), I felt an overwhelming sense of peace and unity. I would often lie with her, and it seemed that we both drifted into a meditative state together. Now I find that my feelings are confirmed by scientific studies done in England. They say that mother and child share periods of meditative sleep until two weeks after the child stops nursing.*

The calm experienced during nursing provides periods of quiet rest for the mother. Giving birth is physically strenuous, and afterward you must respect your body's need for rest. You need good food and relaxation, and so does your baby. If you treat both your baby and yourself with equal gentleness, you will both flourish.

*ICEA News-International Childbirth Association *Spring Quarterly,* March 1970.

11

BEING BORN: LABOR AND BIRTH FROM THE CHILD'S PERSPECTIVE

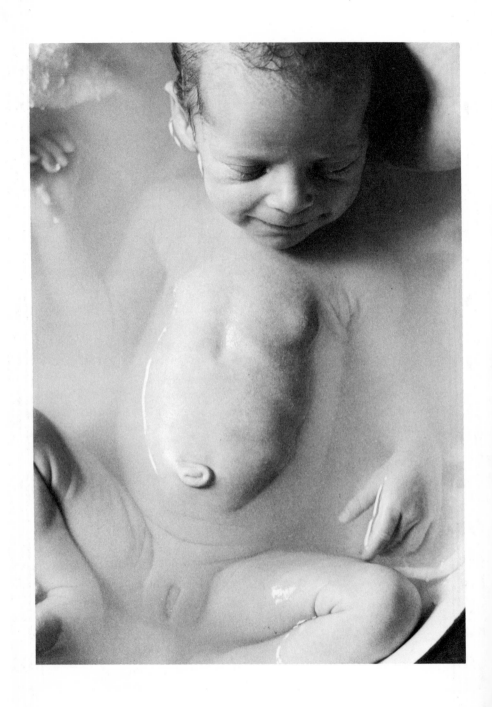

Being Born

To understand the child's experience during labor, at birth, and directly after birth takes some imagination. But every mother who has been present and aware during childbirth can sensitively project what the small creature inside her undergoes.

If we liken the small contractions of the final month to an earth tremor, the contractions of labor must be like a full-scale earthquake. The baby's whole environment closes in on his small body with force. It squeezes, it pushes, it hammers at the child, forcing him slowly down a tunnel. The baby cannot escape the grip of this powerful force. He curls up in a tight ball, his heart beating faster and faster. Then the quaking subsides. There is calm again— but not for long; soon another contraction grips the infant. Again the baby is crushed. The process continues.

The child's endurance is awesome. His head enters the passageway. The force that has gripped the infant not only squeezes, it twists. The small body painfully twists around. The baby's head is like a screw making its way slowly through hard wood. It's difficult to open the passage. It takes force, and the head bears the burden. The head is pushed between the shoulder blades into the chest. As the child struggles to escape, he meets resistance in front and pressure on all sides. The force subsides and then hits more strongly, over and over again. Each time the infant's strength to endure increases. Suddenly the baby's head is released into a flood of light. There is no more pressure on the head. Moments later the body slithers out. For the first time the infant feels the touch of another human, hears the sound of voices, and sees light.

The First Experiences

The kind of experience a child has at this crucial time is the responsibility of mother, father, doctor, and attendants. Dr. Frederick Leboyer, in his wonderful book *Birth without Violence*, has made us aware of and sensitive to the possibilities for a pleasurable entry into the world.

The baby's first cry may be due to the pain of the first breath. If this happens, the child can be calmed by his mother's body and hand. His skin has never been touched. Let the first things to touch it be soft and caressing. (The head, however, does not have to be touched. It is so sensitive from all that pressure.) The room should be dimly lit. The baby has lived in a dark cave; sudden bright lights would be very shocking. The room should be as warm as the mother's body. The cord can wait to be cut. Wait until it stops pulsating, until it is no longer a live part of the baby's body. You can hold your baby before the cord stops beating. It's a long cord and it will reach even if the baby is in your arms or on your stomach.

At this moment, you may want to welcome your baby to the world with some special prayer or ceremony that acknowledges the origin of the soul in God. After the birth of our child, my husband initiated this simple ceremony, which comes from the Hindu tradition: A gold object is dipped in honey, and with it the word *Om* in Sanskrit (written ॐ), the symbol for God, is traced on the child's lips. Gold stands for knowledge and honey for speech. Thus we wished our child a life dedicated to seeking knowledge of God, and the gift of kind and uplifting speech.

After the cord is cut, let your baby nurse if he wishes. The warmth and pleasure of giving and receiving food will make your bond to each other strong. Then allow the father to share in this bond by letting him slowly place his baby in a warm body-temperature bath.

Consciousness at Birth

When a newborn person is cared for in this way, his consciousness is obvious. His eyes are open. He makes contact with the people he first meets. He coos, grunts, smiles.

The research of Dr. Marshall Klaus demonstrates how sensitive and aware newborn infants are. Dr. Klaus has toured the United States showing sound films of newborn babies taken in slow motion. In the films the babies dance and move in perfect time to the rhythm of voices of people who are attempting to communicate with them. They have their own way of saying "Hello"!

Dr. Klaus's work goes far beyond the emotional impact of these films. It also shows significant differences between babies who are born naturally, remaining in contact with their mothers, and those who are kept in hospital nurseries, having minimal contact with their mothers. The "high contact" babies have higher I.Q.'s and are better adjusted throughout the first year of life.*

It is a matter of respect for the human dignity of our child that we treat him with kindness, warmth, and gentleness during the first moments of life.

*See Dr. Martin Richards, "One-Day-Old Deprived Child," *New Scientist,* March 28, 1974.

MANJU'S BIRTH

Our own child was blessed with a perfect birth. Dr. Leboyer's work had not been published in 1973 when Manju was born. We didn't expect our child to be so totally aware. We thought she'd be like a baby kitten, eyes closed, isolated in her own little world.

However, we did think she should be born at home in a calm and loving atmosphere. We knew a doctor, Hector Prestera, a gentle and sensitive man. He agreed to help us. He said, "I'm not an expert," but we knew he had delivered twenty healthy babies at home and never had a woman tear.

It was time for Manju to be born. A few friends who had been singing quietly for hours sat in the room. Hector asked everyone to be still and perfectly quiet.

Her head came out. She was showered by silent vibrations of love from her father, her mother, her doctor, her friends. Hector cleaned her nose and throat. She whimpered and then gurgled. Perfectly healthy, yet without even one cry, she was born.

Her body slithered out. Hector held her to his ear. She was silent. He whispered a mantra in her ear. She listened. Then she was placed in my arms. Even before the cord was cut she looked, eyes wide open, directly into my eyes for several minutes. Then she continued to drink in her new environment. She looked at her dad. Then she looked directly at nearly every person in the room. The cord had now stopped pulsating. She had been born for five to ten minutes. Hector placed her on my stomach and cut the cord. She made only cooing sounds. He placed her back in my arms, and she began to nurse.

It occurred to us then that she was the strongest, most conscious, most mature person in the room. Perhaps it was because she was so new, perhaps because she had become so strong through birth. From that moment it seemed she grew younger rather than older. She seemed to grow from a silent sage into a baby. For months people would tell her, "Little person, you have the face of a wise old man."

Her birth and her being were not an oddity. It's natural for a baby to calmly accept life. All normal infants are strong and clear and conscious. Through the practice of yoga, we can restore our own sense of strength, clarity, and consciousness. Thus we are able to share with our newborn child a simple and perfect joy.

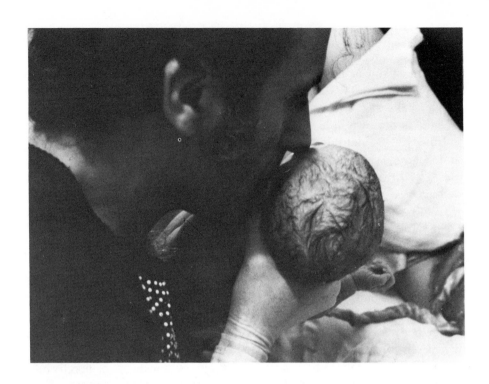

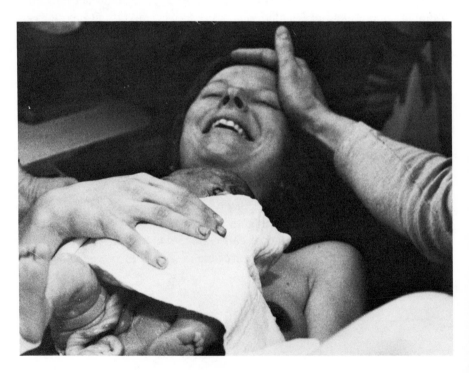

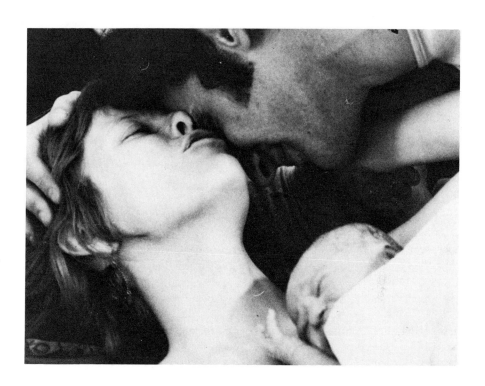

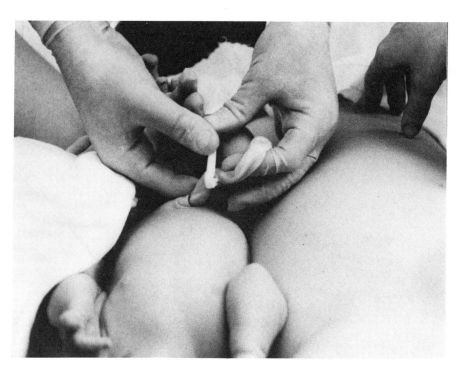

SUGGESTED READING LIST

Arms, Suzanne. *Immaculate Deception*. New York: Bantam, 1975.

Dass, Baba Hari. *Silence Speaks*. Santa Cruz, Calif.: Sri Rama Foundation, 1976.

Dass, Ravi, and Aparna, eds. *The Marriage and Family Book*. New York: Schocken Books, 1978.

Dick-Read, Grantley, M.D. *Childbirth without Fear*. New York: Harper and Row, 1959.

Gaskin, Ina May. *Spiritual Midwifery*. The Farm, Summertown, Tenn.: The Book Publishing Company, 1978.

La Leche League. *The Womanly Art of Breastfeeding*. Franklin Park, Illinois: La Leche League International, 1958.

Lappé, Francis M. *Diet for a Small Planet*. New York: Ballantine, 1975.

Leache, Penelope. *Your Baby and Child*. New York: Alfred A. Knopf, 1978.

Leboyer, Frederick. *Birth without Violence*. New York: Alfred A. Knopf, 1975.

Millinair, Catherine. *Birth: Fact and Legend*. New York: Crown Publishers, 1974.

Nilsson, Lennart. *A Child is Born*. rev. ed. New York: Delacorte, 1977.

Parvati, Jeannine. *Hygieia*. Berkeley, Calif.: A Freestone Collective Book, 1978.

Rosen, Mortimer, M.D., and Rosen, Lynn, Ed.D. *In the Beginning: Your Baby's Brain before Birth*. New York: New American Library, 1975.

Sussman, Vic. *The Vegetarian Alternative*. Emmaus, Pa.: Rodale Press, 1978.

"Vegetarian Mother's Milk is Safer," *New Age Journal,* vol. 4, no. 6 (Dec. 1977) p. 19.